High
Blood Pressure
Demystified

All-in-One Guide with Practical Advice and Support for Hypertension Patients and Their Families

EVERYDAY HEALTH GUIDE – BOOK 2

Dr. K. V. Sahasranam

Copyright

Disclaimer

The information in this book is intended for educational purposes only and is not a substitute for professional medical advice, diagnosis, or treatment. While every effort has been made to ensure accuracy, medical knowledge on hypertension continues to evolve, and readers should consult a healthcare provider for personalized advice.

The patient scenarios included are fictional and meant for illustrative purposes. Any treatments or lifestyle changes discussed should only be considered with professional medical guidance. The author and publishers are not liable for any loss or damage resulting from the use of this information.

I dedicate this book

to my revered teachers of Medicine,

whose guidance instilled in me

the art and science of healing

and the wisdom to know when to intervene

and when to refrain.

My deepest gratitude and respect

are extended to each one of them.

लोका: समस्ता: सुखिनो भवन्तु

Loka samastha sukhino bhavanthu

May all beings everywhere be happy

A Humble Request to the Reader

Thank you for buying and reading this book. May I request your indulgence for one more favor.

I hope you enjoyed reading this book and derived benefit from the various topics discussed.

Kindly give your sincere and valuable Review of this book in the Amazon site. Your rating and candid review will be a great inspiration and encouragement to me.

Please check out my other books given at the end of this book.

Check out my Website at **kvsauthor.com**

You can contact me at my email address

kvsauthor@gmail.com

TABLE OF CONTENTS

Check Out My Books On Amazon

NON-FICTION

How to Face the Challenges while Growing Old
Problems of Elderly Book 1

Old Age Health Challenges and Solutions
Problems of Elderly Book 2

Understanding the Electrocardiogram
Medical Book on ECG

Demystifying Hinduism
Understanding Hinduism Book 1

The Avadhoota – Whispers of Wisdom
Understanding Hinduism Book 2

Daily Musings
Understanding Hinduism Book 3

How to Master Essential Life Skills   Skill sets for
Success Book 1

How to Achieve Professional Excellence   Skill sets
for Success Book 2

FICTION

Tell Me a Story, Grandpa   Short Stories for Children

Grandpa, Tell me More Stories   Short Stories for Children

In Search of a Bridegroom   An Autobiographical Fiction

The Truth Lies Out There   A Family Drama of Suspense

Code Black   A Hospital based Thriller

Diabetes Demystified   Everyday Health Guide Book 1

A Free Gift for the Reader

Here is a FREE Gift for you

Discover The Secrets To A Healthy Heart

<u>Download Your FREE eBook Today!</u>

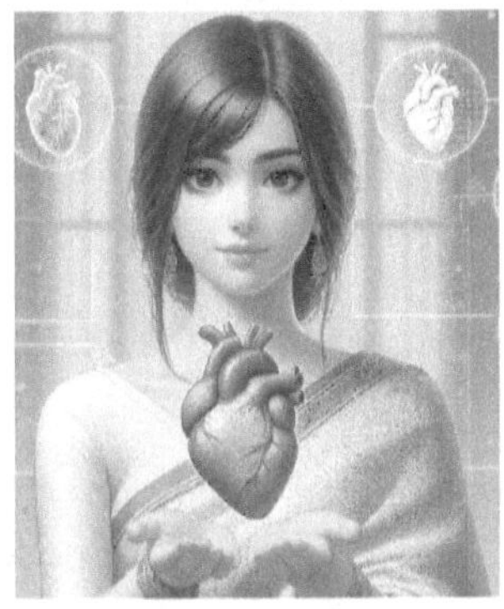

Did you know that heart disease is the leading cause of health problems worldwide? Take charge of your heart health today with my **FREE** eBook, **"Diseases of the Heart."**

Get Your **FREE** eBook Now! **VISIT THE SITE BELOW:**

<u>**https://sahasranam.ck.page/708a4d8aa7**</u>

Or SCAN the QR code given below

About the Author

Dr. K. V. Sahasranam MD, DM, FACC, FCSI, is a distinguished Cardiologist and former Professor of Cardiology at Calicut Medical College, India. With over 45 years of medical practice, he has retired and now resides in the USA. His deep passion lies in educating students and residents, reflected in his book, **"Understanding the Electrocardiogram,"** designed for medical students and physicians, which thoroughly explores the ECG and simplifies its interpretation. Additionally, Dr. Sahasranam offers a comprehensive *3-module course on ECG* through the Udemy platform.

Writing under the pen name *'Sahasranam Kalpathy,'* he has authored 12 more books, spanning both fiction and nonfiction. His works include a series on *'Problems of the Elderly'* (2 books), *'Understanding Hinduism'* (3 books), *'Skillsets for Success'* (2 books), three captivating Fiction novels and two books of Short stories for children.

His first book in the *'Everyday Health Guide'* series' is **"*Diabetes Demystified*"**. This is the second book in the series.

Visit his WEBSITE at: **kvsauthor.com**

Chapter 1 - INTRODUCTION

In this chapter, you will be introduced to the basics of high blood pressure, or Hypertension. We will explore what blood pressure is, how it is categorized, and what defines hypertension. You will learn why it is often referred to as the "Silent Killer" and how it can go unnoticed while causing serious health problems over time. The chapter will also cover the global prevalence of hypertension, key risk factors, and why early detection is crucial for preventing complications. This introduction lays the groundwork for understanding the broader impacts of hypertension on health.

High blood pressure (**HBP**), also known as *Hypertension*, is one of the most prevalent lifestyle diseases worldwide, affecting millions across all age groups. Alongside conditions such as diabetes, obesity, and heart disease, hypertension represents the impact of modern living—characterized by poor diet, sedentary behavior, and stress—on human health. It is often referred to as the *"Silent Killer"* because it can quietly damage the body without causing obvious symptoms. Unlike an acute illness that requires immediate medical attention, high blood pressure often goes unnoticed until it leads to more severe and often catastrophic complications such as heart disease, stroke, or kidney failure.

One of the most concerning aspects of high blood pressure is that it can develop and persist for years without detection. Individuals may feel healthy while their cardiovascular system endures increasing strain. Over time, this silent and gradual process can cause extensive damage to the heart, blood vessels, kidneys, and other vital organs, leading to serious health issues if left unmanaged. For this reason, understanding hypertension is crucial, especially since it is both preventable and manageable in most cases.

Prevalence and Incidence

To understand the scope of hypertension, it is imperative to distinguish between two key epidemiological terms:

Prevalence: *This refers to the total number of people currently diagnosed with hypertension in a population at a given time.*

Incidence: *This refers to the number of new cases of hypertension diagnosed over a specific period, typically one year.*

The prevalence of hypertension varies depending on factors such as age, race, ethnicity, and geographic location. For instance, in the United States, non-Hispanic Black adults have the highest prevalence of hypertension (57.1%) compared to non-Hispanic White adults (43.6%). Age is also a significant factor; about 22.4% of adults aged 18–39 have high blood pressure, but the prevalence rises dramatically with age, affecting 54.5% of adults aged 40–59 and 74.5% of adults aged 60 and older. As per the Center for Diseases control (CDC) 120 million adults in the US have HTN. Almost ½ of the adults in the US have a blood pressure over 130/80 mmHg.

Of the different countries, Africa has the highest prevalence of hypertension, with about 46% of adults aged 25 and above affected. Europe follows closely behind Africa, with about 35-40% of adults suffering from hypertension. In China, the numbers are staggering, with over 270 million people living with hypertension and only 13.8% of people living with HTN have it under control.

India presents a contrasting scenario with its rising urban prevalence of hypertension. In urban areas, approximately 1 in 3 adults (33%) is affected by high blood pressure. Historically, hypertension was less common in rural areas, but this is rapidly changing. With lifestyle shifts, such as increased consumption of processed foods, decreased physical activity, and higher stress levels, rural areas are catching up, reflecting the broader public health challenge that India faces.

Location also plays a role. A study in 2021 showed that the prevalence of hypertension varied across different states in the U.S, from 24.6% in Colorado to 40.6% in Mississippi. Globally also, hypertension is a growing public health issue, with an estimated 1.28 billion adults aged 30–79 affected, according to the World Health Organization (**WHO**). Alarmingly, two-thirds of those with hypertension live in low- and middle-income countries, where healthcare resources are often limited. A significant portion of individuals with hypertension remains untreated or inadequately treated, making it a critical public health challenge.

Public Health Impact of Hypertension

Hypertension has far-reaching consequences not only for individuals but also for healthcare systems and economies. The public health impact of high blood pressure is significant due to the following factors.

Healthcare Costs: Managing hypertension and its associated complications constitutes a substantial portion of healthcare spending globally. This includes direct costs such as medications, doctor visits, and hospitalizations, as well as indirect costs resulting from complications like heart disease, stroke, and kidney failure. In many low- and middle-income countries, these costs can be prohibitive, leading to inadequate treatment and a higher prevalence of complications. In countries like India, where insurance coverage is limited, individuals often have to bear the burden of chronic treatment costs for hypertension. However, government subsidies and insurance coverage are available for hospitalized patients in many cases.

In the United States, hypertension is one of the leading drivers of healthcare expenditure, with billions of dollars spent annually on treatments and hospitalizations.

Lost Productivity: Hypertension also takes a toll on workforce productivity. It can lead to chronic illness, disability, and premature death, all of which contribute to lost workdays and reduced economic output. Individuals with uncontrolled hypertension often require frequent doctor visits, hospitalizations, and ongoing medical care, limiting their ability to work and contribute economically. Furthermore, hypertension-related conditions like heart attacks and strokes can result in long-term disability or death, particularly in working-age adults. This loss of productivity affects not only individual families but also has broader economic implications for society as a whole.

Some Important Technical Terms

Before proceeding further, let us briefly get acquainted with some terms used in this book which are derived from medical terminology.

***Metabolism** refers to the physical and chemical reactions in the body that change food into energy and those that use energy*. They are the sum total of all chemical changes that take place in a cell or an organism. These changes generate energy and produce many other chemical substances that the cells and organisms need to grow, reproduce, and stay healthy. Metabolism also helps get rid of toxic substances from the body.

__Homeostasis__ refers to any automatic process that a living being uses to keep its body steady on the inside while continuing to adjust to conditions outside of the body, or in its environment. The body makes these changes constantly to work and survive. A state of balance among all the body systems is needed for the body to survive and function correctly. *Homeostasis is the ability to maintain a relatively stable internal state that persists despite changes in the world outside.* For example, whether the surrounding temperature rises or falls, the human body remarkably maintains its internal temperature at a steady 37 degrees Celsius (98.6 degrees Fahrenheit). Similarly, the blood's pH is tightly regulated within the range of 7.35 to 7.45, ensuring the stability necessary for vital biochemical processes to occur seamlessly.

__Mortality__ means the rate of death, or the number of deaths occurring within a specific population over a given period of time. It refers to how many people die from a particular disease or condition. In other words, it means the death rate, or the number of deaths in a certain group of people in a certain period of time. Mortality may be reported for people who have a certain disease, live in one area of the country, or who are of a certain gender, age, or ethnic group. Doctors and researchers might discuss the *"mortality rate"* of a disease, meaning how likely someone is to die from that disease.

__Morbidity__ refers to a disease or medical condition that causes illness or injury but does not result in death. It can also refer to the negative effects of a medical treatment or surgery. The physical and psychological impact of a chronic condition, such as decreased quality of life or chronic symptoms is also called morbidity due to that condition. It is the amount of disease within a population. Medical problems caused by a treatment is also referred to as morbidity.

Prognosis *in medical terms means a doctor's prediction about how a disease is likely to develop and what the chances of recovery are for a patient, essentially it is a "forecast" of what to expect with an illness.* It is the likely outcome or course of a disease, the chance of recovery or recurrence. A prognosis is based on the doctor's knowledge of the disease and the patient's individual situation, but it need not always be completely accurate. When giving a prognosis, a doctor will consider things like the severity of the disease, the patient's age and overall health, and the available treatment options. Hence, it indicates the likely outcome or course of the disease - the chance of recovery or recurrence.

Body Mass Index (BMI) *is a measure of body fat based on the height and weight of a person.* It is applicable for adults.

BMI is calculated by dividing the weight (in kilograms) by the square of the height (in meters). It can also be calculated by dividing the weight in pounds by the square of the height in inches multiplied by a conversion faction of 703.

BMI = **Weight (in Kg) ÷**

Height (in meters)^2

BMI = **Weight (in pounds) ÷**

(Height (in inches)^2 $\rbrack \times$ **703**

A general rule of thumb to determine your ideal weight is as follows: subtract 100 from your height in centimeters. The result is your ideal weight in kilograms. For instance, if your height is 160 centimeters (5'4"), your ideal weight would be 160 minus 100, which equals 60 kilograms.

The Purpose of This Book

This book aims to simplify the complex medical concepts related to hypertension and make them accessible to everyone, regardless of medical background. Whether you are a patient, caregiver, or simply someone interested in health, this book will help you understand what hypertension is, why it matters, and how it can be managed effectively.

A key goal of this book is to empower readers with knowledge. Understanding your own health is the first step toward taking control of it. By learning about hypertension and its effects on the body, you will be better equipped to make informed decisions about lifestyle changes, treatments, and medical care. Whether it is through adopting a healthier diet, engaging in regular physical activity, or understanding the role of medications, this book will guide you on how to actively manage your health.

Throughout this book, you will find discussions on Lifestyle Modifications, Pharmacologic interventions, Blood Pressure Monitoring Techniques, and Prevention Strategies. Practical advice and tips will be provided for people living with hypertension, as well as for those caring for loved ones with the condition. By making these concepts easy to understand, the book ensures that everyone can take steps to improve their health and quality of life.

Readers may notice that certain details about hypertension are repeated in various chapters of this book. This repetition is _intentional_, ensuring that even if someone reads only a few chapters, they still receive all the necessary information for a complete understanding. Each chapter is designed to stand alone, allowing readers to engage with specific sections without needing to follow the book in sequence. This approach caters to both casual readers and those looking for comprehensive insights, while also reinforcing key points for better retention.

To help with understanding, many of the technical and medical terms used in the book are explained in brackets in the text itself. The technical terms are given in _italics_. Therefore, a separate glossary is not included at the end. Definitions of terms are _underlined and in italics_.

At the beginning of each chapter, you will find a brief Introductory paragraph that highlights the key points covered. This overview gives the reader a quick snapshot of what to expect, helping the reader get a clear sense of the chapter's content and main themes before diving into the details. At the end of each chapter, I have included a few "_Key Takeaways_" which gives the reader a glimpse of the facts discussed in the chapter.

Additionally, a list of References and recommended reading is appended at the end of the book. This list is for readers who want to seek more detailed academic information regarding hypertension.

Throughout the book, Patient Scenarios illustrate real-life experiences with hypertension, drawn from the author's medical practice. These stories provide examples of practical insights into managing the condition, with the patient names changed to protect privacy. They aim to help readers understand the complexities of hypertension and the importance of proper management. The book includes various figures and tables throughout, designed to help readers grasp concepts more easily. These visual aids have been introduced to present complex details in a simpler, more accessible way.

Towards the end of the book, you will find a chapter on Diet and Nutrition, offering a selection of recipes from both the U.S. and India. While it is impossible to cover every dietary preference, additional reading is recommended for those seeking specific meal plans. A chapter on Resources, Support Groups, and helpful apps offers tools to make managing hypertension easier. The final chapter on Future Directions may seem technologically complex for some readers, but its purpose is to offer a glimpse into potential advancements in hypertension management. It provides insight into emerging treatments and innovative designs that could shape the future of care, giving readers an idea of what to expect in terms of new drugs and therapies.

Finally, while this book focuses on managing hypertension, it also serves as a resource for individuals who do not have high blood pressure but are interested in preventing it or learning how to support others. I hope this book serves as a comprehensive guide to understanding and managing hypertension.

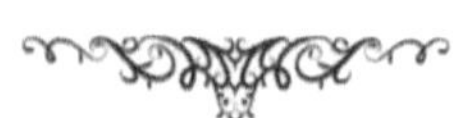

Chapter 2 - HISTORY OF BLOOD PRESSURE MEASUREMENT

The history of high blood pressure, or hypertension, is a fascinating journey that highlights the evolution of medical knowledge and treatment. For centuries, people struggled to understand this condition, which often presented no symptoms but silently damaged the body. Early ideas were crude, involving methods like bloodletting and salt restrictions. However, as our understanding of the human body advanced, so did our approach to hypertension. From the recognition of its link to heart and kidney disease to groundbreaking studies like the Framingham Heart Study, the treatment of high blood pressure has transformed dramatically. This chapter traces the key milestones in the history of hypertension,

Around 129-200 AD, Galen, a Roman physician, proposed that blood was produced in the liver and consumed by the organs, but he did not fully understand the concept of blood circulation. Despite his incorrect theory, Galen's ideas laid the groundwork for later breakthroughs in understanding how the body works.

In 1628, a British physician William Harvey published "*De Motu Cordis*" (On the Motion of the Heart and Blood), where he introduced for the first time the groundbreaking idea that the heart pumps blood in a continuous circuit through the body. This discovery set the stage for comprehending blood pressure. It was a moment of revelation in the field of cardiovascular physiology.

In 1727, Stephen Hales, an English clergyman and scientist, performed the first recorded measurement of blood pressure. He inserted a brass tube into a horse's artery and attached a glass tube nine feet long vertically to it. Hales observed how the blood rose within the tube, thus quantifying arterial blood pressure. The blood rose to a height of 8 feet 3 inches! With every heart beat the top of the column of blood was seen to fluctuate by three inches. This was the first documented record of blood pressure. His innovative experiment marked a pivotal moment in recognizing blood pressure as something measurable and significant.

Soon, a French physiologist Jean Poiseuille made great strides in understanding blood flow. He developed Poiseuille's law, which describes how blood flows through vessels depending on the pressure and resistance it encounters. While not directly related to blood pressure measurement, this work deepened the understanding of how blood pressure affects circulation.

The journey of understanding and treating high blood pressure spans centuries, marked by pivotal discoveries and evolving concepts. Early descriptions of hypertension came from notable figures like Thomas Young and Richard Bright. Richard Bright, in particular, recognized the association between hypertension and kidney disease, laying the foundation for later research into the relationship between the two.

The term "Essential Hypertension," referring to high blood pressure with no identifiable cause, was first introduced by Eberhard Frank in 1911. This condition, which we now know affects the majority of hypertensive patients, remains a major focus of research. The year 1928 saw another significant development when physicians from the Mayo Clinic coined the term "Malignant Hypertension." This referred to severe cases of hypertension that led to damage in vital organs such as the kidneys and the retina of the eye. If left untreated, these patients often faced dire consequences, including strokes, heart failure, or kidney failure, and frequently died within a year of diagnosis.

It is worth noting that even prominent historical figures suffered from severe hypertension. Franklin D. Roosevelt, the 32nd President of the United States, was one such individual. He was under treatment for his condition, but unfortunately, he died in 1945 from complications related to his uncontrolled high blood pressure.

In 1937, Paul Dudley White, a pioneering American cardiologist, reflected the medical thinking of his time when he wrote, *"Hypertension may be an important compensatory mechanism which should not be tampered with, even if we were certain that we could control it."* This viewpoint, which now seems surprisingly incorrect, reflects the belief that high blood pressure, even up to levels of 210/100 mmHg, might actually be *'beneficial'* and therefore did not require intervention. It was only in the 1950s that the medical community recognized the serious dangers posed by untreated hypertension. The concept of hypertension as a 'silent killer' became widely accepted, and the need to manage elevated blood pressure was acknowledged.

The turning point came with the launch of the landmark Framingham Heart Study in 1948. Conducted in the town of Framingham, Massachusetts, and still ongoing today with its third generation of participants, this study revolutionized our understanding of cardiovascular risk factors. It was through this research that the direct link between hypertension, heart disease, and increased mortality was firmly established. The Framingham study provided crucial evidence that high blood pressure is a major contributor to cardiovascular events like heart attacks and strokes.

Early Treatments for Hypertension

The treatment of high blood pressure has a long and curious history. In earlier times, hypertension was known as "Hard Pulse Disease," and treatments were as crude as the understanding of the disease itself. Physicians practiced bloodletting or applied leeches to patients' skin in the belief that lowering the blood volume would reduce blood pressure. Another odd treatment involved injecting *pyrogens*—substances that cause fever—in the hope of lowering blood pressure.

As time progressed, the late 19th and early 20th centuries brought a greater focus on dietary interventions, particularly strict salt restrictions. It was recognized that salt played a role in elevating blood pressure, and extreme salt reduction became a common recommendation for patients with hypertension. However, these methods were only marginally effective.

Modern Treatment and Advances

The modern era of hypertension management began in the 1950s with the advent of oral diuretics. These drugs, by helping the body eliminate excess salt and water, proved to be a significant breakthrough in reducing blood pressure. This was just the beginning of a new approach to hypertension treatment. Over the years, a variety of medications have been developed, including Beta-blockers, ACE inhibitors, Calcium channel blockers, and Angiotensin receptor blockers (ARBs), each targeting different mechanisms involved in blood pressure regulation.

Today, the management of hypertension is highly personalized, with a focus not only on reducing blood pressure but also on addressing the overall cardiovascular risk of the patient. The insights gained from decades of research have transformed what was once thought of as a minor inconvenience into a critical aspect of preventive medicine, saving countless lives worldwide.

Development of the Sphygmomanometer

In 1855, German physiologist Karl von Vierordt created a device designed to track the pulse wave. He called it the *Sphygmograph*. While it could not measure blood pressure directly, it was one of the earliest attempts at creating a non-invasive method to understand the dynamics of blood flow.

Samuel von Basch, an Austrian physician, in 1881 invented the first mercury apparatus to measure the blood pressure. He called it the *Sphygmomanometer*. The word "sphygmomanometer" is derived from the Greek words "*Sphygmos*" and *Manometer*. *Sphygmos* means 'beating of the heart' or 'pulse'. '*Manometer*' is a 'device used for measuring pressure or tension'. This was the first instrument that allowed for non-invasive measurement of blood pressure. It marked the beginning of practical tools for doctors to assess a patient's blood pressure.

The modern era of blood pressure measurement began with an internist, Scipione Riva-Rocci in 1896. He introduced an inflatable cuff connected to a mercury column, which allowed for a more accurate measurement of systolic blood pressure. This method quickly became the standard due to its reliability and ease of use.

In 1905, a Russian surgeon, Nikolai Korotkoff made a groundbreaking advancement by identifying specific sounds—later named '*Korotkoff sounds*'—heard through a stethoscope while measuring blood pressure. By listening to these sounds as the cuff slowly deflates, both systolic and diastolic pressures can be measured. This remains the foundation of modern blood pressure measurement. Even today, the Korotkoff sounds heard with a stethoscope are used while measuring the blood pressure in patients.

Mercury sphygmomanometers became the gold standard throughout the 20th century. Their accuracy and reliability made them the primary method of blood pressure measurement in hospitals and clinics worldwide. However, as concerns over mercury toxicity grew, many countries began phasing out these devices in favor of safer alternatives.

Modern Techniques / Devices

<u>Aneroid Sphygmomanometers</u>: *Aneroid* (using no liquid) sphygmomanometers emerged as a safer alternative to the mercury apparatus. These devices use a mechanical dial to display pressure readings. They are more portable and widely used in various healthcare settings but require regular calibration to maintain accuracy.

<u>Electronic and Automated Devices</u>: Electronic devices that measure blood pressure using oscillometric methods detect the oscillations in the arterial wall as the cuff deflates. These monitors have become popular for home use due to their convenience, but in some cases, they may not be as accurate as manual devices.

<u>Ambulatory Blood Pressure Monitoring</u> (**ABPM**): Ambulatory blood pressure monitoring is a diagnostic test that measures blood pressure over a period of time while a patient continues their normal activities. It is considered one of the most accurate way to measure blood stressure and diagnose hypertension and often used by physicians to detect hourly and night time changes in blood pressure. ABPM allows for continuous blood pressure measurement over 24 hours, providing a

detailed profile of a person's blood pressure throughout the day and night. This method is particularly useful in identifying conditions like white coat hypertension, where blood pressure spikes in a clinical setting but remains normal elsewhere. These will be discussed in detail later. [See Chapter 5 on *Blood Pressure Measurement*].

Home Blood Pressure Monitoring (**HBPM**): The availability of home blood pressure monitors has helped patients to manage their health by tracking their blood pressure on a regular basis. Studies have shown that home monitoring can significantly improve blood pressure control by allowing earlier intervention and more consistent follow-up. The patient becomes aware of the changes in his blood pressure and adheres to his treatment. [See Chapter 5 on *Blood Pressure Measurement*].

Recent Advances

Wearable Blood Pressure Monitors: Wearable devices, like smartwatches that can measure blood pressure, are becoming more common and popular. These allow continuous monitoring without the need for a traditional cuff. However, current technology is still being refined to ensure accuracy and reliability. These are not used by doctors to monitor treatment in patients.

Telemedicine and Digital Health: The integration of blood pressure monitoring with telemedicine platforms has made it possible for patients to share real-time data with healthcare providers. This allows for better remote management of conditions like hypertension and has proven especially useful during the COVID-19 pandemic.

The use of telemedicine has become very popular during the pandemic.

Future Directions

Emerging Technologies: Researchers are developing non-invasive methods to continuously monitor blood pressure using newer technologies like Photoplethysmography (**PPG**) and Pulse Transit Time (**PTT**). These techniques aim to revolutionize blood pressure management by providing patients with more accurate and convenient monitoring tools.

Challenges and Considerations

Calibration and Accuracy: No matter how advanced the technology is, ensuring accuracy remains a crucial aspect of blood pressure monitoring. Devices should be regularly calibrated and validated against clinical standards to guarantee reliable readings.

Access and Affordability: Despite all these technological advancements, access to reliable blood pressure monitors remains a challenge in many parts of the world. Affordable, easy-to-use devices are essential to help manage hypertension on a global scale.

Blood pressure measurement has come a long way, from Hale's glass tube experiment on a horse to today's digital, portable monitors. The continuous evolution of technology aims to improve accuracy, accessibility, and convenience, helping millions of people manage their health more effectively.

Key Takeaways:

- *Hypertension was first described in detail by physicians like Thomas Young and Richard Bright, who linked it to kidney disease.*
- *The term "Essential Hypertension" was introduced in 1911 to describe high blood pressure with no identifiable cause.*
- *"Malignant Hypertension," a severe form of the condition causing organ damage, was defined in 1928 by Mayo Clinic physicians.*
- *Early treatments for hypertension included bloodletting, leeches, and strict salt restriction, though they were largely ineffective.*
- *Modern understanding of hypertension evolved through key studies like the Framingham Heart Study, which highlighted its role in cardiovascular disease and mortality.*
- *The treatment of hypertension significantly improved in the 1950s with the discovery of diuretics and the development of various effective medications.*
- *Untreated high blood pressure was once thought to be harmless, but today it is recognized as a major risk factor for heart disease, stroke, and kidney failure.*

Chapter 3 - HEART AND THE CIRCULATORY SYSTEM

Before considering the specifics of high blood pressure, it is important to understand the heart and circulatory system, as these are at the core of the body's blood pressure regulation.

Structure and Function of the Circulatory System

The circulatory system's primary role is to deliver blood to various parts of the body, ensuring the supply of oxygen and nutrients while removing waste products. The heart, a remarkable muscular organ, lies at the center of this system. Despite its small size—approximately that of a closed fist, weighing around 9-12 ounces (250-350 grams)—the heart pumps blood throughout the body, operating tirelessly throughout one's life.

Located slightly to the left inside the chest cavity, the heart is shielded by the breastbone and spine in front and behind. It contains four chambers: two upper chambers known as the *Atria* (singular: *Atrium*) and two lower chambers called the *Ventricles*. The atria receive blood from all parts of the body, while the ventricles pump it out to reach all parts.

Blood enters the right atrium (**RA**) from two large veins: the *Superior Vena Cava* (**SVC**), which collects blood from the upper body, and the Inferior Vena Cava (**IVC**), which collects blood from the lower body. On the left side, oxygenated blood from the lungs enters the *Left Atrium* (**LA**) via four *Pulmonary Veins*. From the LA blood enters the *Left Ventricle* (**LV**) which pumps this oxygen-rich blood into the *Aorta*, the body's largest artery. The aorta distributes the blood to the rest of the body through its various branches. Meanwhile, the *Right Ventricle* (**RV**) pumps *deoxygenated* (oxygen-depleted) blood into the pulmonary artery, which carries it to the lungs for oxygenation.

Arteries, Veins, and Capillaries

Blood vessels play a vital role in this process. Arteries, such as the aorta, transport oxygen-rich blood from the heart to various parts of the body. The walls of the arteries contain smooth muscles that allow vessels to expand (*dilate*) and contract (*constrict*) as blood flows through them. In contrast, veins return oxygen-depleted, carbon dioxide-rich blood back to the heart. Once in the lungs, oxygen from the air we breathe in is absorbed into the blood, while carbon dioxide is expelled as we exhale.

The inner lining of the arteries and veins are composed of a sheet of cells called the *Endothelium*. The endothelium releases a protein called *Endothelin* which caused blood vessels to become narrow (*constrict*).

As arteries move away from the heart, they branch into increasingly smaller vessels, culminating in tiny *Capillaries*. These hair-thin vessels have walls so thin that oxygen and nutrients can pass into surrounding tissues, while carbon dioxide and metabolic waste move from the tissues into the blood. The capillaries then converge into veins, which carry the waste-laden blood back to the heart. This circulation cycle ensures the continuous exchange of vital substances throughout the body.

Heart Valves: Ensuring One-Way Blood Flow (Fig 1)

Within the heart, blood flows in only one direction, thanks to a system of valves that act like gates. Between the atria and ventricles are two main valves: the *Tricuspid Valve* (**TV**) on the right side, and the *Mitral Valve* (**MV**) on the left side. These prevent backflow of blood into the atria. Similarly, the *Aortic Valve* (**AV**) and *Pulmonary Valve* (**PV**) prevent blood from flowing back into the ventricles after being pumped out to the body or lungs through the aorta and the pulmonary artery respectively. This system ensures a smooth, forward flow of blood through the heart and circulatory system.

The Heartbeat: The Body's Electrical System

The heart beats approximately 70 times per minute (60 -100) in a healthy adult, driven by a small but powerful structure called the *Sinus Node*. Located in the upper right atrium, the sinus node functions like a natural pacemaker, generating regular electrical *impulses* (signals) that trigger the heart to contract. These impulses are transmitted throughout the heart via specialized fibers, causing the heart muscle to contract in unison.

The heart works continuously throughout life, with only brief milliseconds of rest between beats. Remarkably, it beats about 100,000 times each day—an incredible testament to its endurance.

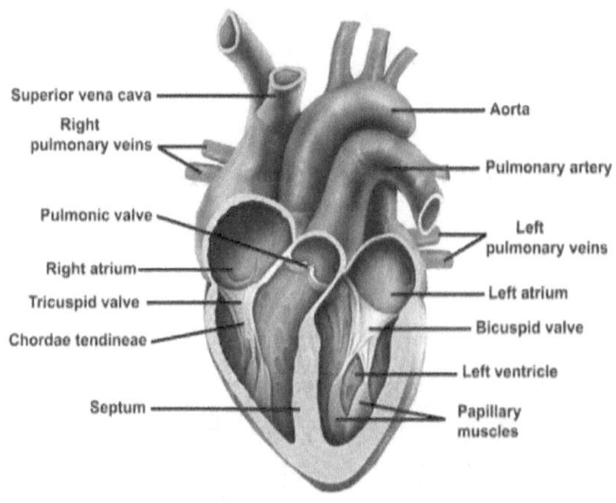

Fig 1. Structure of the Heart

The Heart's Vital Role

The heart's primary function is to pump oxygen-rich blood to every part of the body, while also collecting carbon dioxide and waste products. The carbon dioxide is expelled through the lungs during exhalation, and the waste products are filtered out by the kidneys, then excreted as urine. The heart also plays a critical role in maintaining the body's blood pressure, pumping approximately 5.5 liters (1.5 gallons) of blood every minute.

Despite its relentless work, the heart requires its own supply of oxygen and nutrients. This is delivered via three small arteries, called *Coronary Arteries*, which arise from the aorta and encircle the heart. A blockage in these arteries can lead to a heart attack, one of the most serious cardiovascular events.

The Two Circulations: Pulmonary and Systemic   [Fig 2]

The circulatory system is divided into two circuits: *Pulmonary Circulation* and *Systemic Circulation.*

Pulmonary Circulation: Blood enters the right ventricle and is pumped into the pulmonary artery, which transports it to the lungs. There, the blood is oxygenated before returning to the left atrium via the pulmonary veins. This short loop of circulation, responsible for oxygenating blood, is referred to as the *'Lesser circulation.'*

Systemic Circulation: Oxygenated blood from the left ventricle enters the aorta and is carried throughout the body via its numerous branches. As blood flows through organs and tissues, it delivers oxygen and nutrients, collecting carbon dioxide and waste products in return. This deoxygenated blood is then brought back to the right atrium by the superior and inferior vena cava. This much longer route is known as the *'Greater circulation.'*

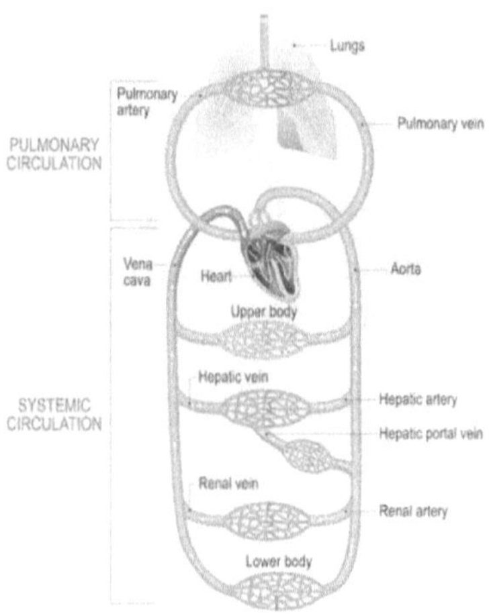

Fig. 2. Pulmonary & Systemic Circulation

Coronary Arteries: Lifeblood of the Heart

Two key branches of the aorta supply blood to the heart muscle - the right and left coronary arteries. The right coronary artery supplies the right side of the heart, while the left coronary artery splits into two branches—the *Left Anterior Descending Artery* and the *Left Circumflex Artery*—to supply the left side. Without proper blood flow through these arteries, the heart muscle cannot function effectively, potentially leading to heart disease.

Some Fascinating Facts

- The human heart is about the size of the individual's closed fist.
- *It beats around 100,000 times per day.*

- *The average adult heart beats 60-100 times per minute, while a newborn's heart beats much faster at 100-160 beats per minute.*
- *The heart pumps about 1.5 gallons (5.5 liters)of blood per minute, amounting to over 2,000 gallons per day.*
- *Blood travels about 12,000 miles throughout the body daily—roughly four times the distance across the United States.*
- *The body contains approximately 60,000 miles of blood vessels, enough to circle the Earth twice.*

By understanding the heart and circulatory system, we gain insight into how blood pressure is regulated and how it affects the health of these vital structures.

Chapter 4 - CAUSES, PATHOPHYSIOLOGY AND RISK FACTORS

High blood pressure is a condition where the force of blood against the walls of the arteries is consistently too high. This chapter explores the key causes and underlying mechanisms that contribute to hypertension. Factors like genetics, lifestyle habits (diet, lack of exercise), and certain medical conditions play a role in its development. The pathophysiology involves complex systems in the body, such as the Renin-Angiotensin-Aldosterone System (RAAS), nervous system, and blood vessel function, which, when disrupted, lead to sustained high blood pressure. Understanding these causes helps in better managing and preventing hypertension.

High Blood Pressure (**HBP**), medically known as *Hypertension*, is a condition that affects millions worldwide. It is a significant risk factor for heart disease, stroke, kidney failure, and other serious health conditions. Understanding the causes and underlying mechanisms is crucial for managing and preventing the long-term effects of hypertension. This chapter provides a detailed look at the two main types of hypertension—*Primary* and *Secondary*—and describes the physiological processes involved, as well as key risk factors contributing to its development.

Pathophysiology means the abnormal changes in body functions that occur due to a disease and its causes.

Primary vs. Secondary Hypertension

Hypertension can be broadly classified into two categories: *Primary (Essential) Hypertension* and *Secondary Hypertension*. Each type has distinct causes and implications for treatment.

Primary (Essential) Hypertension

Primary hypertension is the most common form, accounting for about 90-95% of all cases. It develops gradually over many years and has no identifiable cause. This form of hypertension is typically diagnosed during routine blood pressure screenings or after complications arise.

HTN is often called the *"Silent Killer"* because it can be asymptomatic for many years. The diagnosis of HTN is usually made after elevated blood pressure readings are consistently observed. Patients may experience symptoms such as headaches, dizziness, or nosebleeds, but these tend to appear only after the condition becomes severe. Majority of patients have no symptoms.

Pathogenesis

Pathogenesis is the process whereby a disease or disorder develops. The exact mechanisms behind primary hypertension are not fully understood, but it is believed to result from a combination of genetic, environmental, and lifestyle factors. Several hypotheses have been proposed to explain its development:

Renin-Angiotensin-Aldosterone System (**RAAS**) Dysregulation: This system is a set of hormones produced by the kidney and the adrenal gland. When these hormones are overactive, it makes the body retain too much salt and *constrict* (tighten, narrow) the blood vessels. This leads to increased blood pressure that remains high.

Overactive Sympathetic Nervous System: The *Sympathetic Nervous System* (**SNS**) is that part of the nervous system which regulates the involuntary functions in the body like the beating of the heart, movements in the intestines and breathing. When this part of the nervous system is too active, it causes the blood vessels to narrow and make the heart beat faster. This increases blood pressure.

Endothelial Dysfunction: The *endothelium* (lining of blood vessels) normally produces substances that help blood vessels relax. In HTN, the production of these substances is reduced, and this lining does not function properly, so the blood vessels stay narrow, and this makes it difficult for blood to flow smoothly.

Inflammation and Oxidative Stress: Long-term, low-level inflammation and damage to blood vessels can make them stiff and narrow, which also increases blood pressure.

Secondary Hypertension

Secondary hypertension accounts for 5-10% of all cases. Unlike primary hypertension, secondary hypertension arises due to an identifiable and often treatable underlying cause.

Causes

Kidney Disease: Chronic kidney disease (**CKD**) and *Renovascular Hypertension* (narrowing of the arteries to the kidneys) are common causes. The kidneys play a crucial role in blood pressure regulation, and any impairment can lead to hypertension.

Endocrine Disorders:

- Primary Aldosteronism (Conn's Syndrome): Excess *Aldosterone* (a salt-retaining hormone) production by the adrenal gland leads to sodium retention and potassium loss, raising blood pressure.

- Cushing's Syndrome: Overproduction of *Cortisol* (stress hormone) by the adrenal gland increases blood pressure.

- Pheochromocytoma: A rare tumor of the adrenal gland that releases catecholamines, such as *Adrenaline* (a hormone), causing episodic or persistent hypertension.

- <u>Obstructive Sleep Apnea</u> (**OSA**): Repeated interruptions in breathing occurring during sleep activate the sympathetic nervous system, raising blood pressure. This can be caused by obesity, heart and kidney failure, reduced thyroid gland function and many more disorders.

- <u>Medications</u>: Certain drugs, such as NSAIDs, Oral contraceptives, Corticosteroids, and Decongestants used for cough, can induce or exacerbate HTN.

- <u>Other Causes</u>: Conditions like *Coarctation of the Aorta* (a congenital narrowing of the main artery arising from the heart) or thyroid disorders (*hyperthyroidism* and *hypothyroidism*) can also cause secondary hypertension.

Diagnosis and Management:

It is vital to identify secondary hypertension because treating the underlying cause can often resolve or significantly improve blood pressure control. Diagnostic approaches include blood tests, imaging, and sometimes more specialized tests, such as measuring renin and aldosterone levels or conducting sleep studies.

Physiology of Hypertension Development

Physiology is the branch of biology that deals with the normal functions of living organisms and their parts. It explains the way in which a living organism or bodily part functions. It describes the chemistry and physics behind basic body functions.

Hypertension results from complex interactions between various systems in the body, including the blood vessels, kidneys, heart, and nervous system. These systems work together in a coordinated manner to regulate blood pressure. Dysfunction in any of them can lead to elevated levels.

Over time, high blood pressure leads to changes in the structure of blood vessels. The arterial walls become thicker, and the *lumen* (the inside cavity of the artery) narrows. This process, known as *vascular remodeling*, increases the resistance that blood encounters as it flows through the body. This raised resistance keeps blood pressure high.

The endothelium plays an essential role in maintaining blood vessel tone by releasing substances like nitric oxide which relax the blood vessels thereby prevent it from becoming narrow. When the BP is low, it produces substances which *constrict* (narrow down) the blood vessels thereby raising the BP. In hypertensive patients, the function of the endothelium is affected causing the blood vessels to remain constricted and this contributes to high blood pressure.

Chronic low-grade inflammation in the body is increasingly recognized as a factor leading to HTN. Substances released in the body during inflammation can damage blood vessels, leading to stiffening and narrowing.

As already discussed, the RAAS plays a central role in blood pressure regulation. When blood pressure drops, the kidneys release *Renin*, a hormone, which starts a chain reaction that produces substances that narrow down the blood vessels. These substances also stimulate the adrenal glands to secrete aldosterone, which causes the kidneys to retain sodium and water in the body. Renin also causes another substance Angiotensin II to form. These lead to increased blood pressure.

Overactivity of the Sympathetic Nervous System

The brain has a center which controls blood pressure. It signals all the BP regulators in the body through the *Autonomic Nervous System* which has two parts – *Sympathetic Nervous System* (**SNS**) and the *Parasympathetic Nervous System* (**PNS**). The SNS signals increase blood pressure whereas the signals from the PNS lower BP back to normal.

The SNS is responsible for the body's "fight or flight" response, which includes increasing heart rate and constricting blood vessels. In hypertension, this system can be overactive, causing sustained vasoconstriction and elevated heart rate, both of which raise blood pressure.

Stress, obesity, insulin resistance, and sleep apnea are known to increase sympathetic activity, leading to higher blood pressure. The SNS also interacts with the RAAS, amplifying the hypertensive effects.

The kidneys are responsible for regulating sodium balance in the body. In HTN, the kidneys may struggle to excrete the excess sodium. Being unable to do so leads to water retention and increased blood volume, which raises blood pressure.

In healthy individuals, when blood pressure rises, the kidneys excrete more sodium and retain sodium when the blood pressure falls. In hypertensive patients, however, this mechanism is impaired, meaning higher pressures are required to induce sodium excretion, further perpetuating high blood pressure.

Genetic Predisposition

Hypertension often runs in families, with genetic factors contributing to its development. Variations in genes can increase the risk of developing high blood pressure.

Metabolic Factors

Insulin resistance, where the cells resist the action of insulin is a hallmark of *Metabolic Syndrome*. This is closely linked to hypertension. Metabolic syndrome is characterized by *obesity, high fasting blood sugar, high blood lipids, insulin resistance and HBP.*

Obesity is a major risk factor for hypertension. *Adipose tissue* (fat) produces substances which can influence blood pressure by affecting appetite, metabolism, and vascular health. In the year 2000, about 365,000 deaths in the United States were associated with being overweight or obese. 1 in 5 children in developed countries are found to be overweight or obese. 4 of 10 adults are overweight and this ratio is expected to be 1 in 2 by 2030.

Risk Factors

Several factors like lifestyle, genetics and environment contribute to the risk of developing hypertension. These can be classified as *Modifiable* (those that can be changed) and *Non-modifiable* (those that cannot be changed). Most of the lifestyle factors are modifiable whereas family history and genetics are non-modifiable.

Lifestyle Factors

Dietary Influences

Excessive salt consumption is a significant risk factor for hypertension, particularly in people who are salt-sensitive. Potassium helps balance sodium's effects. A low-potassium diet can contribute to higher blood pressure. Diets high in processed foods and unhealthy fats increase the risk, while diets rich in fruits, vegetables, and whole grains (e.g., the DASH diet) help lower blood pressure. [See Chapter 16 on *Diet and Nutrition*].

Physical Inactivity

Sedentary behavior is linked to an increased risk of hypertension. Regular physical activity strengthens the heart and reduces vascular resistance, helping to lower blood pressure.

Alcohol and Tobacco Use

Excessive alcohol consumption and smoking are both risk factors for hypertension. Smoking, in particular, causes immediate *vasoconstriction* (narrowing of blood vessels) and long-term damage to the arteries.

Stress

Chronic stress can raise blood pressure by stimulating the sympathetic nervous system and increasing the production of stress hormones, such as cortisol.

Genetic Factors - Family History

A family history of hypertension significantly increases one's risk. Genetic factors are estimated to account for 30-50% of the variability in blood pressure among individuals.

Thus we find that HTN is a highly complex condition influenced by a range of causes, including genetic, lifestyle, and environmental factors. The distinction between primary and secondary hypertension is critical in guiding treatment and management. Hence, understanding the underlying mechanisms of hypertension helps in identifying appropriate interventions and lifestyle changes to control the condition. By recognizing and addressing the various risk factors, individuals can take steps to prevent or manage high blood pressure, reducing the risk of serious health complications such as heart disease, stroke, and kidney failure.

Key Takeaways:

- *Hypertension occurs when the force of blood against artery walls is consistently high, putting strain on the heart and blood vessels.*
- *Key causes include genetics, poor diet, lack of physical activity, and medical conditions like kidney disease.*
- *Overactivity in systems like the Renin-Angiotensin-Aldosterone System (RAAS) and the Autonomic nervous system can lead to high blood pressure by increasing fluid retention and narrowing blood vessels.*

- *Blood vessel dysfunction and chronic inflammation also contribute to hypertension by making arteries stiff and less able to relax.*
- *Understanding the causes and mechanisms of hypertension is crucial for effective management and prevention.*

Chapter 5 - BLOOD PRESSURE MEASUREMENT

Understanding how blood pressure is measured is essential for managing and diagnosing hypertension. Blood pressure reflects the force of blood against the walls of your arteries and is recorded as two numbers: Systolic and Diastolic. Accurate measurement is key, whether in a doctor's office, at home, or using advanced devices. In this chapter, we will explore the importance of proper technique, the different methods used, and how to interpret your readings to ensure a clear understanding of this vital health indicator.

Blood pressure is one of the most critical health metrics, often referred to as a silent indicator of overall cardiovascular well-being. For many, understanding blood pressure may seem like a daunting task, but it is crucial for preventing severe health issues, such as heart disease, stroke, and kidney failure. We shall discuss some basic facts about blood pressure, how it is measured, and what those numbers mean in practical terms.

Basics of Blood Pressure

Blood Pressure (BP) is the force exerted by circulating blood against the walls of arteries. It plays a vital role in maintaining the flow of blood through the circulatory system, ensuring that oxygen and essential nutrients reach the body's tissues while waste products are removed. Without proper blood pressure regulation, essential organs like the heart, brain, and kidneys can suffer damage.

Blood pressure is measured in *millimeters of mercury* (**mmHg**) and is typically recorded as two numbers.

Systolic Blood Pressure (SBP) represents the peak pressure in the arteries when the heart's lower chambers (Ventricles) contract and push blood into the circulation. It is the first number recorded in a blood pressure reading, such as the **120** in a reading of 120/80 mmHg. The higher the systolic pressure, the greater the strain on your arteries, especially if it is consistently elevated.

Diastolic Blood Pressure (DBP) reflects the pressure in the arteries when the heart is at rest between beats, allowing it to refill with blood. This is the second number in a blood pressure reading, such as the **80** in 120/80 mmHg. It indicates the minimum pressure exerted on your arteries, which still requires attention, as persistently high diastolic readings also indicate cardiovascular risks.

Pulse Pressure *is the difference between systolic and diastolic pressures.* A normal pulse pressure (usually around 40 mmHg) indicates healthy arterial function. Higher values may signal arterial stiffness, a sign of aging or cardiovascular disease.

Blood pressure serves as an important health marker. Normal blood pressure (around 120/80 mmHg) ensures that all organs receive adequate blood supply. Both elevated and low readings can indicate health issues. Persistently high blood pressure, or *Hypertension*, significantly raises the risk of life-threatening conditions like heart disease, stroke, and kidney damage. On the other hand, low blood pressure, or *Hypotension*, can cause dizziness, fainting, and in severe cases, shock. Hence, keeping the blood pressure within the normal range is important in maintaining long-term health.

Measurement of Blood Pressure.

Accurately measuring blood pressure is critical in diagnosing hypertension and assessing cardiovascular risk. Let us discuss how to ensure correct blood pressure readings. - Three goals for the initial evaluation of blood pressure are:

1. Accurate measurement of BP
2. Assessment of the patient's overall cardiovascular risk
3. Detection of Secondary forms of HTN

Preparation for Measurement:

To achieve the most accurate blood pressure reading, it is essential to follow certain preparatory steps.

- Ensure that you or the patient are comfortably seated for at least 5 minutes before taking a measurement.
- Avoid caffeine, smoking, or exercise for at least 30 minutes prior to checking the blood pressure, as these can temporarily raise blood pressure levels.
- Sit with your back supported, feet flat on the floor, and legs uncrossed. The arm being measured should rest at heart level, preferably resting on a table and the cuff should be placed on bare skin (not over clothing) on the upper arm.
- One should remain silent during the recording.
- Using the right-sized cuff is important for accuracy. A cuff that is too large or too small can lead to false readings. The cuff should fit snugly around the upper arm, with the lower edge about an inch above the elbow. The cuff should surround at least 80% of the circumference of the arm.

Manual Devices: These are traditional devices that require using a stethoscope to listen for *Korotkoff sounds* (the sounds of blood flow) as the cuff deflates. Manual devices tend to be more accurate when used properly, but they require training. The Mercury sphygmomanometer and the Aneroid sphygmomanometer are the two devices used for manual readings.

Automated Devices: These are widely used in homes and clinics because they are simple to operate.

While convenient, it is important to use validated models as some may be less accurate, especially in individuals with irregular heartbeats.

<u>Measuring Blood Pressure manually.</u>

- Inflate the cuff to 20-30 mmHg above the point where you no longer feel the radial pulse at the wrist.
- Slowly deflate the cuff (about 2-3 mmHg per second) while listening for the Korotkoff sounds using the stethoscope placed over the brachial artery at the elbow.
- Record the systolic pressure when the Korotkoff sounds first appear and the diastolic pressure when the sounds disappear.

<u>Measuring with an Automated device.</u>

- Follow the instructions given on the device carefully. Ensure that the cuff is placed correctly and remain still and quiet during the measurement. Automated devices will provide both systolic and diastolic values, often with the pulse rate displayed.
- Blood pressure can fluctuate due to various factors like stress or physical activity. Taking two or more readings, spaced 1-2 minutes apart, and averaging them, can give a more reliable result. If the difference between the two readings is significant, a third reading may be necessary.

The readings should be taken in both arms and the arm giving the higher reading is chosen for the subsequent readings.

Special Considerations

White Coat Hypertension:

Many people experience higher-than-usual blood pressure when measured in a clinical setting in the doctor's office due to anxiety, a condition known as 'White Coat Hypertension'. For these individuals, home or Ambulatory blood pressure monitoring (**ABPM**) might provide more accurate results.

Masked Hypertension:

The reverse of white coat hypertension, 'Masked hypertension' refers to normal readings in a clinical setting but higher readings at home or in everyday environments. Regular home monitoring can help diagnose this condition.

Resistant Hypertension

Resistant hypertension refers to high blood pressure that remains elevated despite the use of three or more antihypertensive medications, including a diuretic, taken at optimal doses. This condition affects a small but significant portion of hypertensive patients and signals an increased risk of cardiovascular complications such as heart attacks, strokes, and kidney damage.

Resistant hypertension may result from underlying factors like obesity, excessive salt intake, or other medical conditions, such as sleep apnea or kidney disease. In some cases, it may be attributed to secondary causes of hypertension, such as hormonal imbalances or medications that interfere with blood pressure control.

Effective management of resistant hypertension involves identifying and addressing these underlying causes, optimizing medication regimens, and implementing lifestyle changes, including weight loss, a low-sodium diet, and regular physical activity. For patients who do not respond to these measures, advanced treatments, such as device-based therapies or referral to a hypertension specialist, may be necessary.

Recognizing and managing resistant hypertension is crucial to prevent serious health outcomes and improve the overall quality of life. Regular follow-ups, careful monitoring, and a comprehensive approach are key to successful control of this challenging condition.

Interpreting the Numbers

Once the blood pressure reading is taken, it is essential to understand what those numbers mean for your health.

Blood Pressure Categories

Blood pressure is classified into several categories based on systolic and diastolic values. This is summarized in Table 1.

Normal Blood Pressure: A blood pressure reading of less than 120/80 mmHg is considered normal. Individuals with normal blood pressure have a low risk of cardiovascular complications.

Elevated Blood Pressure: Systolic blood pressure between 120-129 mmHg and diastolic pressure of 80 mmHg or lower falls under this category. While not classified as hypertension, elevated blood pressure indicates a higher risk of developing high blood pressure over time.

Prehypertension: Systolic blood pressure between 120 – 139 mmHg and diastolic pressure between 80 – 89 is called *Prehypertension.*

Hypertension Stage 1: A systolic pressure ranging from 130-139 mmHg or a diastolic pressure between 80-89 mmHg is classified as Stage 1 hypertension. This stage requires lifestyle changes and possibly medication to prevent further progression.

Hypertension Stage 2: A systolic pressure of 140 mmHg or higher or a diastolic pressure of 90 mmHg or higher indicates Stage 2 hypertension. This is a more severe stage that typically requires a combination of medications and lifestyle interventions to manage.

Blood Pressure	Values - (mmHg)
Normal	< 120/80
Elevated	120 – 129 / 80
Prehypertension	120-139 / 80-89
Hypertension Stage 1	130 – 139 / 80 – 89
Hypertension Stage 2	≥ 140 / 90

Table 1 : Blood Pressure Categories

A systolic pressure of 180 mmHg or higher or diastolic pressure of 120 mmHg or higher is a medical emergency and requires immediate treatment. Symptoms like severe headache, shortness of breath, chest pain, or blurred vision may accompany this condition. It is vital to seek medical attention if you consistently record high readings, especially if they reach hypertensive crisis levels. Uncontrolled high blood pressure can damage vital organs and lead to life-threatening events like a heart attack or stroke.

Various factors can influence blood pressure readings, sometimes leading to misinterpretation. Hence, we should be aware of these and record the blood pressure when the individual is relaxed. Some of these factors are as follows.

External Factors:

- Caffeine, Nicotine, and Alcohol can raise blood pressure temporarily.

- Blood pressure naturally rises during exercise but should return to normal after resting. Hence, BP should be recorded only 30 minutes after physical activity.

- Anxiety and stress can lead to temporarily elevated readings of BP.

- Medications can increase BP. NSAIDs, Oral contraceptives, Chemotherapy drugs and antidepressants are known to increase BP.

Physiological Factors:

- As people age, arteries naturally become stiffer, often leading to higher systolic pressure.

- Excess weight strains the cardiovascular system, increasing blood pressure.

- Conditions like diabetes, kidney disease, and sleep apnea can contribute to hypertension.

Home Blood Pressure Monitoring

Home blood pressure monitoring (**HBPM**) plays a crucial role in managing hypertension and assessing treatment effectiveness. By tracking blood pressure over time, patients can provide valuable data to their healthcare providers, helping to fine-tune treatment strategies.

HBPM or self-monitored BP (**SMBP**) measurement is now coming up in a big way to overcome many of the obstacles in hypertension management. It overcomes many of the disadvantages encountered in the office BP measurement by traditional methods. It is reliable, easy to use, and of late affordable monitors are available. It can be used in patients who are not well educated and is easily taught to the patient or to the care giver. In the present era, when telemedicine is becoming more popular, HBPM is of utmost importance in proper follow-up and medication titration.

Some points to be remembered while recording BP at home are:

- Select a validated, automatic monitor for home use. Ensure it is calibrated regularly to maintain accuracy.
- For those managing hypertension, taking readings at least once a day at the same time is recommended.
- Recording the date, time, and reading for each measurement can help both you and your doctor identify patterns and assess the effectiveness of your treatment.

The main advantages of HBPM are:

- o Multiple readings are possible
- o Avoids the white coat effect
- o Reproducible
- o Better predicts the chances of complications than office BP recording
- o Can diagnose White coat hypertension, Masked hypertension, Labile hypertension, and Paroxysmal hypertension (See later for details)
- o Patients understand the treatment better and hence compliance to treatment is increased
- o More measurements can be obtained during a limited period
- o HBPM data correlate better with daytime ABPM
- o Telemonitoring allows remote monitoring by the health care professional
- o Cost effective.

However, we should understand that HBPM is not without some limitations. Let us discuss some of these.

- ✓ Some devices are found to be inaccurate. Choice of a proper device is hence very important. A study in 2011 reported that almost 30% of the devices were inaccurate. Hence, the choice of a proper device is of paramount importance.
- ✓ The cuff placement can affect the accuracy of the reading. Care should be taken to position the cuff on the arm properly.
- ✓ Less suitable in subjects with a large arm circumference as an appropriate cuff may not be available. One should ensure that the cuff used is proper for the individual.
- ✓ HBPM may not be accurate in patients with an irregular pulse.

- ✓ HBPM may not be accurate when there is considerable vascular stiffening.
- ✓ In some patients, it may induce undue anxiety and excessive monitoring unnecessarily. Some thus may become obsessed with their BP recording.
- ✓ Risk of self-medication and change of medications without the doctor's guidance (self-treatment) is always a concern. Patients should be told not to change (reduce or increase) their medications without their physician's advice.
- ✓ Lack of *nocturnal* recording. This means that the blood pressure during night cannot be recorded using HBPM. For this the ABPM is ideal.
- ✓ Not reimbursable by insurance in most countries.

My personal advice to patients is to bring the device to the clinic with them initially and for one or two subsequent visits where they are asked to record the BP in my presence. Any faults in tying the cuff or measurement is corrected then. The BP is then measured in the office using the office device by the doctor or nurse. This fairly validates the accuracy of the patient's device. This is a simple method to ensure correct readings and to inculcate a sense of confidence in the patient. It also corrects any mistakes the patients may be doing while recording their BP.

Ambulatory Blood Pressure Monitoring

The recording of BP in the office depends on many factors. Though simple, the measurement of BP is fraught with many drawbacks due to lack of standardization, improperly validated equipment, wrong cuff size, improper training of personnel taking the BP, inadequate rest for the patient before recording, smoking prior to the measurement, etc.

The Ambulatory Blood Pressure Monitoring (**ABPM**) provides the advantage of measuring the BP several times an hour for 24 hours and thus gives us recording during the normal activities during the day in addition to the *diurnal* (happening during day and night time) variations in reading. The BP can also be divided into the daytime, night-time, and a graph of the diurnal variation plotted to give the highs and lows during the 24-hour period.

It is seen that a '*non-dipping pattern*' (not decreasing) of BP reading and *nocturnal* (night time) hypertension both are associated with increased cardiovascular morbidity and mortality. Approximately 70% of the population show a *dip* (decrease) in the BP by about 10% at night compared to about 30% of the population who have *non-dipping* patterns. Their BP may remain the same as day or even be higher during the night-time. Thus, the results of the ABPM can help the clinical management of the patient by predicting the CV risk and helping to time the dose of drug administration.

It is a cost-effective diagnostic and prognostic investigation that can be used in day-to-day practice. However, it is an underutilized investigation, especially by the community physicians. For a valid and reliable assessment, there should be at least 20–25 readings spread out over 24 hours.

Indications for Ambulatory Blood Pressure Monitoring

The main indications where ABPM can be of immense use are as follows:

- Labile hypertension – where there are abrupt and unexpected changes in BP during the day, classically seen in pheochromocytoma (paroxysmal hypertension). [See Chapter 9 on *Labile Hypertension*].
- True resistant hypertension --where the BP is not controlled even with optimal doses of three antihypertensive drugs are used one of which should be a diuretic.
- White coat hypertension – where the patient exhibits a higher BP reading in the clinical setting but does not do so in other settings as in his home.
- Masked hypertension – where the BP recorded in the office is normal, whereas it is high when recorded in other settings such as his home or during ABPM.
- Suspected autonomic dysfunction - when the patient has symptoms of *postprandial* (after a meal) hypotension and heart rate variability.
- Screening for obstructive sleep apnea.
- Hypotensive symptoms when a patient is on treatment.
- To identify circadian time of medication administration i.e. the best time to administer the medication.

Advantages of Ambulatory Blood Pressure Monitoring

The main practical advantages of ABPM over the office BP measurement in the management of high BP are as follows:

- o Multiple recordings are obtained over a 24-hour period.
- o It measures the diurnal variations in BP.
- o It measures the BP and pulse rate during the routine daily activities of the patient.
- o It helps in the diagnosis of white coat hypertension and masked hypertension which may be misdiagnosed based on office recordings alone.

ABPM has given a better correlation with damage to target organs like heart, kidney, eye and brain.

Disadvantages of Ambulatory Blood Pressure Monitoring

The ABPM is not totally devoid of disadvantages. A few of these are given below.

- ✓ In many cities and countries, it is a costly investigation.
- ✓ Limited availability of equipment.
- ✓ Disruption of daily activities and sleep and discomfort when the bladder inflates.
- ✓ There are lesser number of long-term studies about ABPM.

A novel idea in the ABPM is the 1-hour recording of the BP using an ABPM device measured every 5 minutes. The patient is kept in a quiet room in the health center avoiding walking, smoking, or eating. This is being compared with the routine office BP measurement to note whether there is any advantage of this novel method.

Blood pressure measurement is a simple yet essential tool for monitoring cardiovascular health. Understanding what the numbers mean and taking steps to maintain healthy levels can significantly reduce your risk of heart disease, stroke, and other complications. With accurate measurement techniques and consistent monitoring, patients can take control of their blood pressure and, by extension, their overall health.

Key Takeaways

- *Blood pressure is the force exerted by circulating blood on the walls of the arteries.*
- *Systolic pressure represents the pressure during heart contractions, while diastolic pressure measures pressure between beats when the heart is at rest.*
- *Blood pressure is measured in millimeters of mercury (mmHg) and is expressed as systolic over diastolic (e.g., 120/80 mmHg).*
- *Accurate measurement is crucial and can be affected by factors like improper cuff size, body position, stress, and recent activity.*
- *The manual method using a sphygmomanometer and stethoscope is the gold standard for clinical blood pressure measurement.*

- *Automatic digital monitors are widely used for home monitoring but may be less accurate than manual measurements if not used correctly.*
- *Ambulatory Blood Pressure Monitoring (ABPM) and Home Blood Pressure Monitoring (HBPM) provide valuable data for assessing blood pressure variations over time and outside clinical settings.*
- *Ambulatory Blood Pressure monitoring has many advantages and a few disadvantages. However, some of the advantages surpass the disadvantages.*
- *A single blood pressure reading is not enough to diagnose hypertension; repeated readings over time are essential for accurate diagnosis.*
- *White coat hypertension (elevated readings in a clinical setting) and Masked hypertension (normal readings in a clinical setting but high at home) highlight the importance of monitoring in various settings.*
- *Understanding blood pressure readings and ensuring consistent, proper technique is vital for managing and diagnosing hypertension effectively.*

Chapter 6 - SYMPTOMS AND SIGNS OF HYPERTENSION

Hypertension, often called the "Silent Killer," typically presents no obvious symptoms, making it challenging to detect without regular monitoring. However, in more severe cases or during hypertensive crises, individuals may experience headaches, dizziness, blurred vision, or palpitations. This chapter discusses these warning signs as untreated high blood pressure can lead to serious complications like heart attacks, strokes, and kidney failure. This chapter outlines the common symptoms of hypertension, when to seek medical help, and emphasizes the importance of routine blood pressure checks to ensure early diagnosis and management.

Hypertension is a condition that can go unnoticed for many years due to its lack of obvious symptoms.

However, as it silently wreaks havoc on the body, it can manifest through various warning signs. The common symptoms, the reasons hypertension often has no symptoms, and the critical signs that necessitate immediate medical attention are discussed here. The mechanism by which these symptoms occur have also been explained briefly. Through understanding these elements, individuals can become more vigilant in detecting and managing high blood pressure.

Symptoms *of a disease are physical or mental changes that a person experiences that indicate they may have a disease or condition.* Symptoms are sensations that the person with the disease can feel but that cannot be seen by others or measured such as pain or fatigue.

Signs *of a disease are abnormalities that can be observed or measured during a physical exam or lab test and indicate that a person may have a disease or condition.* E.g. fever, inflammation, skin color changes.

Common Symptoms of HTN

While most individuals with hypertension experience no noticeable symptoms, there are some key warning signs that may indicate elevated blood pressure. Being aware of these can prompt timely medical intervention and prevent long-term damage.

Headaches One of the most commonly reported symptoms of hypertension, though not always present, is headache. Hypertensive headaches are often described as dull, throbbing, or persistent, typically occurring in the morning when blood pressure is higher.

The location is often generalized, but patients may feel discomfort at the back of the head or neck. While these headaches are more closely associated with hypertensive crises or severe hypertension, they serve as an important indicator when present.

When blood pressure is high, it can increase the pressure inside the head, leading to irritation and stretching of the sensitive areas in the brain, which can cause headaches. Changes in blood flow may also contribute to this discomfort. However, it is important to understand that mild to moderate high blood pressure does not always cause headaches. This is why it is important to check your blood pressure regularly, even if you feel fine.

Dizziness   Another symptom often reported by patients with hypertension is dizziness. This can range from a sensation of lightheadedness to full-blown *Vertigo* (feeling of spinning) or an unsteady feeling. Dizziness may occur as a result of fluctuating blood pressure, especially in cases of labile hypertension, where blood pressure swings dramatically.

This is due to the reduced blood supply to the inner ear or part of the brain which is concerned with maintaining our posture and balance. It can also be a side effect of antihypertensive medications, particularly those that relax blood vessels or lower blood pressure too rapidly. Although dizziness alone is not always a cause for alarm, it becomes more concerning when it leads to falls or accidents, particularly in older adults who are more susceptible to injuries.

Thomas, a 34-year-old businessman from Tamil Nadu, led a busy life that left little room for health concerns. Fond of rich food, he gradually gained weight, which he dismissed as a consequence of his lifestyle. However, when he began experiencing breathlessness after climbing a flight of stairs, he realized something was amiss. Initially, he ignored the symptoms, attributing them to fatigue. But as his shortness of breath worsened, he finally sought medical attention.

Upon examination, his physician discovered his blood pressure was alarmingly high at 160/116 mmHg. Further tests revealed that Thomas' kidney function and blood parameters were within normal ranges, but his ECG showed signs of left ventricular hypertrophy, later confirmed by an echocardiogram. The physician diagnosed him with Stage 2 hypertension and advised immediate lifestyle changes. Thomas was started on antihypertensive medications and placed on a weight reducing diet. In addition, a graded exercise regimen was recommended to improve his fitness.

Determined to regain control of his health, Thomas followed his doctor's advice diligently. Within four months, he shed nine pounds, and his blood pressure stabilized at a healthy 130/76 mmHg. Feeling lighter and more energetic, he incorporated 30 minutes of playing badminton daily into his routine. Regular home monitoring of his blood pressure became part of his new, healthier lifestyle.

Blurred Vision   Hypertensive retinopathy, a condition caused by prolonged high blood pressure damaging the blood vessels in the eyes, can lead to blurred vision. These visual disturbances occur when the blood vessels in the retina become thickened, narrowed, or torn, reducing the retina's ability to function properly.

Patients may report episodes of transient blurred vision or more persistent visual problems. Severe or prolonged hypertension can lead to more serious eye complications, including permanent vision loss. Regular eye exams and blood pressure management are crucial for preventing such outcomes. [See Chapter 15 on *Complications of Hypertension*].

Nosebleeds (*Epistaxis*) High blood pressure can weaken or rupture small blood vessels, particularly in the nose, leading to nosebleeds. While nosebleeds are not a very common symptom of hypertension, they may indicate poorly controlled blood pressure in some patients

The exact cause involves increased pressure in the tiny blood vessels in the nasal passages, making them more prone to breaking. Recurrent or severe nosebleeds should prompt an evaluation of blood pressure levels to rule out uncontrolled hypertension or other causes such as disorders of blood clotting.

Palpitations Some patients with hypertension may experience palpitations, characterized by a sensation of the heart pounding, fluttering, or skipping beats. These may occur due to the heart working harder to pump against the resistance created by high blood pressure. Palpitations can also be linked to *Arrhythmias* (irregular heart beat), such as *Atrial Fibrillation*, which is more common in individuals with hypertension.

While occasional palpitations are often harmless, they should not be ignored and should be evaluated to ensure that they are not a sign of a more serious condition, such as heart failure or coronary artery disease (**CAD**).

Fatigue and Weakness Hypertension, especially when severe or long-standing, can lead to feelings of fatigue and weakness. These nonspecific symptoms occur as the heart and vascular system are under constant strain, requiring the body to work harder to maintain normal function. This increased workload can cause weariness, reduced physical stamina, and even mental exhaustion.

Fatigue can also be a side effect of certain blood pressure medications, especially Beta-blockers, which can slow the heart rate and lower energy levels. Though these symptoms are not exclusive to hypertension, they can significantly impair daily activities and overall quality of life if left unaddressed.

Chest Pain (Angina) While chest pain is not typically a direct symptom of hypertension, it can be indicative of associated cardiovascular conditions, such as Coronary artery disease (**CAD**) or hypertensive heart disease. Patients may experience tightness, pressure, or pain in the chest, especially during physical exertion or emotional stress.

Chest pain should always be treated as a medical emergency, as it may signal an acute coronary syndrome, such as a heart attack, or a hypertensive crisis. Chest pain is due to decrease in blood being supplied to the heart. Immediate medical attention can help prevent life-threatening complications.

Why Hypertension Often Has No Symptoms

One of the most dangerous aspects of hypertension is its symptomless nature. Despite causing significant damage to the body over time, many individuals with high blood pressure are unaware of their condition until it is detected during a routine check-up or after a serious cardiovascular event, such as a heart attack or stroke occurs.

The majority of individuals with hypertension exhibit no symptoms, earning it the moniker *"Silent Killer."* Without regular blood pressure monitoring, it is easy for people to overlook the condition and continue their lives unaware of the potential danger lurking within them.

Hypertension never develops suddenly. It typically develops gradually over many years. The cardiovascular system can adapt to higher pressures, allowing the body to function without noticeable changes for long periods. This slow progression makes it difficult to recognize when blood pressure has risen to dangerous levels. By the time symptoms such as headaches or chest pain occur, significant damage may have already been done to the heart, kidneys, brain, and blood vessels.

Without routine medical check-ups, many individuals remain undiagnosed and untreated for years, allowing HTN to continue damaging their organs. Studies suggest that as many as *one-third* of people with high blood pressure may be unaware of their condition, increasing their risk of complications like heart attack, stroke, and kidney disease.

The best way to prevent the silent progression of HTN is through regular screening. Simple blood pressure checks, especially in high-risk populations, can detect elevated blood pressure before symptoms appear. Public health campaigns have focused on raising awareness about the importance of screening, emphasizing that even asymptomatic individuals should have their blood pressure checked regularly.

When to Seek Medical Attention

<u>Warning Signs That Require Immediate Care</u>

Certain symptoms, while not exclusive to hypertension, may indicate a more serious issue, such as a hypertensive crisis or the onset of complications. Immediate medical attention is required when these signs appear.

Hypertensive Crisis

A *"Hypertensive Crisis"* occurs when blood pressure spikes dramatically, typically above 180/120 mmHg, posing an immediate risk of organ damage. Symptoms of a hypertensive crisis can include:

- Severe headaches

- Chest pain

- Shortness of breath

- Visual disturbances

- Confusion

- Loss of consciousness

This is a medical emergency, requiring urgent treatment to prevent life-threatening complications like stroke, heart attack, or acute kidney injury. Rapid intervention, including medications to quickly lower blood pressure, is critical. [See Chapter 15 on *Complications of Hypertension*].

Chest Pain and Shortness of Breath

Chest pain and shortness of breath may be signs of a heart attack or other serious cardiovascular conditions.

Chest pain that radiates to the arm, jaw, or back, particularly when accompanied by difficulty breathing, should be treated as a medical emergency. These symptoms warrant immediate evaluation to rule out *Myocardial Infarction* (heart attack) or heart failure.

Severe Headache and Neurological Symptoms

A sudden, severe headache, often described by the patient as *"the worst headache of my life,"* combined with neurological symptoms like weakness, numbness, or difficulty speaking, can signal a stroke or *Hypertensive Encephalopathy*. These symptoms require urgent medical care to prevent permanent brain damage.

Blurred Vision and Eye Pain

Sudden vision changes, including blurred vision, eye pain, or the appearance of floaters or flashing lights, may suggest *Hypertensive Retinopathy* or optic nerve damage. Immediate ophthalmologic evaluation is necessary to prevent permanent vision loss.

Signs of Heart Failure

Unexplained shortness of breath, especially when lying flat or during exertion, along with swelling in the legs, ankles, or abdomen, can indicate heart failure. These symptoms should prompt a thorough evaluation and treatment to prevent worsening heart function.

Severe Anxiety and Palpitations

Intense anxiety, restlessness, and palpitations may accompany a hypertensive crisis or reflect a panic attack exacerbated by high blood pressure. Seeking medical help is important to differentiate between an anxiety episode and a hypertensive emergency.

Persistent Nosebleeds and Fatigue

Frequent nosebleeds, combined with fatigue and weakness, may signal poorly controlled or severe hypertension. A medical consultation is essential to adjust treatment and prevent further complications.

Hypertension, though often symptomless, can have serious consequences if left undiagnosed and untreated. Understanding the common symptoms, the silent nature of the disease, and the warning signs that require immediate medical attention is crucial for both patients and caregivers. Regular monitoring, lifestyle changes, and timely treatment are key to managing high blood pressure and reducing the risk of life-threatening complications.

Key Takeaways

- *Hypertension is often asymptomatic, earning it the nickname "Silent Killer," making regular blood pressure monitoring essential.*
- *Common symptoms of hypertension include headaches, dizziness, blurred vision, palpitations, nosebleeds, and fatigue, but they usually occur in more severe cases.*
- *Hypertensive crises, characterized by extremely high blood pressure (above 180/120 mmHg), can present with severe headaches, chest pain, shortness of breath, and confusion, and require immediate medical attention.*
- *Long-term uncontrolled hypertension can lead to serious complications such as heart disease,*

stroke, kidney damage, and vision loss, even if no symptoms are present early on.

- *Routine screening and early detection are crucial for preventing damage caused by undiagnosed hypertension and improving long-term health outcomes.*

Chapter 7 - MANAGEMENT OF HYPERTENSION:

NON-PHARMACOLOGIC APPROACHES

Hypertension, or high blood pressure, can often be effectively managed without medications through lifestyle changes and natural approaches. In this chapter, we explore non-pharmacologic strategies such as adopting heart-healthy diets like the DASH and Mediterranean diets, increasing physical activity, managing stress, and integrating alternative therapies like yoga and meditation. By making these lifestyle modifications, individuals can lower their blood pressure and improve their overall heart health, often reducing the need for medication while empowering themselves to take control of their condition naturally.

The good news about hypertension is that it is highly manageable, and many individuals can control their blood pressure effectively without relying solely on medication. Let us discuss the non-pharmacologic approaches to managing hypertension, focusing on lifestyle modifications, alternative therapies, and patient education. By following these strategies, patients can lower their blood pressure, improve their overall health, and potentially reduce the need for medications.

Collaborating with your healthcare provider to determine your ideal blood pressure goal is crucial. Generally, a target of less than 130/80 mm Hg is recommended for most individuals. However, your doctor may adjust this target depending on your age, overall health, and risk factors. Regular monitoring of your blood pressure at home can also help track progress and alert you to any changes that may need medical attention.

Beyond just focusing on blood pressure numbers, it is essential to set goals related to your daily habits, particularly in the areas of diet, physical activity, and stress management. These lifestyle changes are fundamental in managing hypertension, and small, achievable targets, such as walking 30 minutes a day or cutting down on salt intake, can lead to significant improvements over time.

Setting goals is important but sticking to them can be challenging. It is normal to face obstacles, but with the right strategies and mindset, you can maintain adherence to the lifestyle changes required to manage hypertension. Common barriers like lack of time, motivation, or external pressures can derail progress. Family support is important to help achieve these goals.

Lifestyle Modifications

One of the most effective ways to manage hypertension without medication is through lifestyle changes. These modifications not only reduce blood pressure but also promote general well-being.

Dietary Interventions

Diet plays a central role in managing hypertension. Certain dietary patterns have been shown to significantly lower blood pressure and reduce cardiovascular risk.

DASH Diet (<u>Dietary Approaches to Stop Hypertension</u>):

The DASH diet is one of the most well-researched dietary interventions for reducing blood pressure. It emphasizes the consumption of fruits, vegetables, whole grains, and low-fat dairy products while reducing sodium intake. Studies have demonstrated that the DASH diet can lower systolic blood pressure by 5-6 mmHg and diastolic pressure by 3 mmHg, particularly when combined with reduced sodium intake. The diet promotes foods rich in potassium, calcium, and magnesium, which are important for regulating blood pressure. It also limits saturated fats, cholesterol, and sweets. The DASH diet encourages reducing sodium intake to less than 2,300 mg per day. For individuals with hypertension, further reductions to 1,500 mg per day have been shown to yield even greater blood pressure improvements. [See Chapter 16 On *Diet and Nutrition*].

Mediterranean Diet: (Fig.1)

The Mediterranean diet is another heart-healthy dietary pattern, rich in whole foods, healthy fats (particularly olive oil), fish, nuts, and vegetables. Studies show that the Mediterranean diet is associated with lower blood pressure and a reduced risk of cardiovascular diseases. This diet emphasizes healthy fats, fiber-rich vegetables, and antioxidant-laden fruits, contributing to overall vascular health. Incorporating Mediterranean principles into daily meals is simple, involving increased consumption of olive oil, nuts, fish, and vegetables while reducing processed foods. [See Chapter 16 on *Diet and Nutrition*].

Weight Management:

Excess weight, especially abdominal fat, increases the risk of hypertension. Losing weight can lead to significant reductions in blood pressure. Effective weight management involves reducing calorie intake, practicing portion control, and choosing nutrient-dense foods. Research indicates that losing even 5-10% of body weight can lead to a noticeable reduction in blood pressure, improving overall cardiovascular health.

Physical Activity

Regular physical activity is an essential component of hypertension management. Exercise helps improve vascular health, reduce inflammation, and lower blood pressure levels over time.

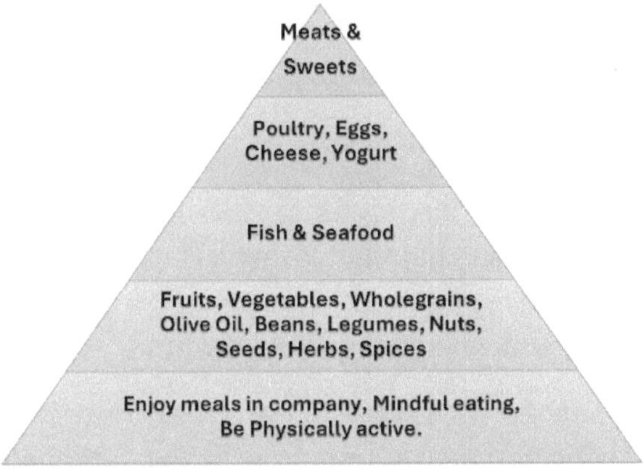

Fig. 1. Mediterranean Diet

Aerobic activities like walking, cycling, jogging, and swimming are particularly effective at lowering blood pressure. These exercises enhance cardiovascular fitness and improve the elasticity of blood vessels. Resistance exercises, when performed safely, can complement aerobic activities. They improve muscle tone, contribute to weight loss, and enhance overall fitness. Experts recommend at least 150 minutes of moderate-intensity exercise per week or 75 minutes of vigorous-intensity exercise.   Physical activity leads to improved blood flow, reduced stress hormone levels, and enhanced *endothelial* (the inner lining of blood vessels) function, all of which contribute to lower blood pressure. [See Chapter 17 on *Prevention of Hypertension*].

Exercise and Blood Pressure Control:

Following exercise, many people experience an acute reduction in blood pressure, known as Post-exercise Hypotension. This benefit can last for hours, helping to regulate blood pressure over the long term. Individuals who maintain a regular exercise routine enjoy lasting improvements in blood pressure control and overall cardiovascular health.

Stress Management

Stress is a significant, often overlooked, contributor to high blood pressure. Chronic stress causes the body to release hormones like cortisol and adrenaline, which elevate blood pressure.

When the body perceives stress, it activates the sympathetic nervous system, leading to *vasoconstriction* (narrowing of blood vessels) and an increase in blood pressure. Studies have shown that individuals with high levels of perceived stress have a higher incidence of hypertension and difficulty controlling their blood pressure.

Stress Reduction Techniques:

Mindfulness techniques, such as meditation and focused breathing, reduce stress by calming the nervous system. *Progressive Muscle Relaxation* is a technique which involves tensing and relaxing different muscle groups, reducing overall physical tension and promoting relaxation.

Cognitive Behavioral Therapy (**CBT**) is a structured form of psychological therapy that helps individuals identify and change negative thought patterns contributing to stress.

Simple daily practices, such as deep breathing, meditation, and ensuring work-life balance, can help manage stress and lower blood pressure. Research shows that stress management techniques improve blood pressure control and reduce cardiovascular risks.

Yoga

While lifestyle modifications form the cornerstone of hypertension management, alternative therapies like yoga and meditation can play a significant role in reducing stress and improving blood pressure.

Yoga combines physical postures, controlled breathing, and meditation, making it a holistic approach to managing both the mind and body. It helps improve muscle strength, flexibility and balance.

Certain yoga poses (*Asanas*) are designed to promote relaxation and improve circulation. *Pranayama* is a controlled breathing technique that reduces sympathetic nervous system activity, calming the body and lowering blood pressure.

Research consistently shows that yoga, when practiced regularly, can reduce both systolic and diastolic blood pressure.

Hatha Yoga is a gentle form of yoga which is ideal for beginners and those with hypertension, focusing on posture alignment and relaxation. Combining yoga with mindfulness enhances its effects on blood pressure, reducing both physical and mental stress.

Meditation

Meditation is a powerful tool for managing stress, which, in turn, helps control blood pressure. Various forms of meditation are effective in reducing blood pressure. Various forms of meditation are described.

Mindfulness Meditation is a practice that focuses on awareness of the present moment, reducing stress and improving overall well-being. *Transcendental*

Meditation involves the repetition of a mantra to calm the mind and reduce stress-related hypertension. *Loving-Kindness Meditation* is a practice that fosters compassion and emotional well-being, indirectly benefiting cardiovascular health. It is also known as *Metta meditation*. This type of meditation is based on ancient Buddhist traditions.

Numerous studies show that regular meditation reduces blood pressure by decreasing sympathetic nervous system activity and stress hormone levels. Meditation practices, when sustained over time, contribute to better blood pressure control, especially for individuals with mild hypertension.

Acupuncture

Acupuncture, a key component of traditional Chinese medicine, has gained attention for its potential in managing hypertension. Acupuncture is believed to influence blood pressure by modulating the autonomic nervous system, reducing stress, and releasing endorphins. Although the evidence is mixed, some studies suggest that acupuncture can help lower blood pressure in certain individuals. It is most effective when used as part of a comprehensive treatment plan and not as a standalone treatment for high blood pressure.

Engaging in enjoyable activities, whether it is reading, gardening, or spending time with loved ones, can also help manage stress and lower blood pressure. Poor time management can lead to stress, which can exacerbate hypertension. Learning to prioritize tasks, set boundaries, and learning to say 'No' can reduce the pressures that contribute to elevated blood pressure both in the office and out of office circumstances.

Herbal Remedies

Herbal supplements are widely used in alternative medicine for managing various conditions, including hypertension. Known for its cardiovascular benefits, garlic has been shown to have mild blood pressure-lowering effects. Drinking hibiscus tea may reduce systolic blood pressure, according to some studies. Hibiscus tea is a caffeine-free herbal tea made from the dried calyces of the hibiscus plant, also known as *Hibiscus sabdariffa*. It has a tart, fruity flavor and can be enjoyed hot or iced. Some studies show that hibiscus tea can help lower blood pressure. It contains antioxidants which help to protect against harmful substances generated in the body called *'free radicals'* which can damage cells in the body. Hibiscus tea may not be suitable for everyone.

Coenzyme Q10 is an antioxidant and is believed to help lower blood pressure, though research is still ongoing. While some herbal remedies show promise, it is crucial for patients to consult healthcare providers before using them, as these supplements can interact with medications.

Patient Education

Knowledge is power. By understanding hypertension and actively participating in its management, patients can significantly improve their health outcomes. Patients should be educated about what hypertension is, its causes, and how it affects the body. Regular blood pressure monitoring and awareness of personal risk factors are key to managing the condition.

Key Takeaways

- *The DASH and Mediterranean diets are highly effective in lowering blood pressure. Reducing sodium intake, increasing consumption of fruits, vegetables, whole grains, and healthy fats like olive oil can significantly help manage hypertension.*
- *Even modest weight loss of 5-10% of body weight can lead to meaningful reductions in blood pressure.*
- *Engaging in at least 150 minutes of moderate-intensity aerobic exercise per week, along with strength training, improves cardiovascular health and helps control blood pressure.*
- *Reducing stress through techniques such as mindfulness meditation, deep breathing, and cognitive-behavioral therapy can lower blood pressure by controlling the body's stress response.*
- *Yoga, meditation, acupuncture, and some herbal remedies may have mild to moderate effects on blood pressure control, complementing lifestyle modifications.*
- *Educating patients about hypertension and encouraging regular self-monitoring of blood pressure helps them take an active role in managing their condition.*
- *Developing a tailored plan with achievable goals for diet, exercise, and stress reduction can lead*

to sustained improvements in blood pressure and overall heart health.

- *Engaging family members and utilizing community or digital resources for guidance and motivation can reinforce adherence to lifestyle changes.*

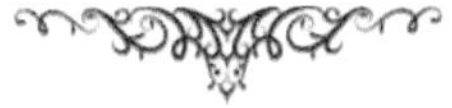

Chapter 8 - MANAGEMENT OF HYPERTENSION:

PHARMACOLOGIC APPROACHES

In this chapter, we explore the pharmacologic approaches to managing hypertension, a key aspect of controlling high blood pressure when lifestyle changes alone are not enough. Medications play a vital role in reducing blood pressure, preventing complications like heart attack, stroke, and kidney damage. In this chapter we will discuss different classes of blood pressure medications, how they work, and why doctors may choose one drug over another. Understanding these treatments can help you work with your healthcare provider to find the best strategy for long-term blood pressure control and overall health.

Hypertension, commonly known as high blood pressure, is one of the most prevalent chronic conditions worldwide. If left untreated, it can lead to serious complications such as heart disease, stroke, and kidney failure. Fortunately, several pharmacologic treatments are available to help manage hypertension effectively. This chapter discusses the various types of antihypertensive medications, their mechanisms of action, and how they are used to manage blood pressure.

Some of the axioms followed in using medications for hypertension are discussed below in brief. These help the patient to stick to their medication schedule in order to obtain optimal control of their blood pressure. Some of these guidelines and tips are:

- ✓ It is wise to start a medication that is inexpensive, having minimal side effects.
- ✓ A medication taken once a day is preferable.
- ✓ Always, the medication is started with lowest dose and gradually stepped up.
- ✓ A second drug of a different class, acting in a different way is added if the BP is not controlled with one drug.
- ✓ If a drug is not tolerated, a drug belonging to a different class is substituted.
- ✓ When heart disease, kidney disease, diabetes etc., are present in addition, a different class of medications are given.
- ✓ Take the medication at a fixed time daily, preferably when you are at home.
- ✓ Using a plastic pill box with compartments for each day of week is convenient. You will not forget or skip the medication.

✓ If you are forgetful, set alarm or use an app like *Medisafe* or *EveryDose*.
✓ If you forget or fail to take a dose DO NOT double next dose.
✓ Always understand the side effects of the medications you are taking by asking your doctor.
✓ If you find any change in BP when taking readings at home, do not change the medications. Ask your doctor.

Medications to Treat Hypertension

Several classes of medications are prescribed to manage hypertension. The choice of medication depends on the patient's health profile, the underlying conditions, and how effectively the medication controls blood pressure. Let us discuss them in brief.

Diuretics

Diuretics, commonly known as 'water pills,' are often the first line of treatment for hypertension. The word diuretic is derived from the Greek word *'diourein'*, meaning "to urinate". They cause the kidneys to produce more urine. Hence the name. They help the body eliminate excess salt and water. This results in a decrease in blood volume and, in turn, lowers blood pressure. There are three main types of diuretics used in managing hypertension:

<u>Thiazide Diuretics</u>   The medications Hydrochlorothiazide and Chlorthalidone belong to this category. They are often the first-choice medication for most patients with HTN and is particularly effective in older adults. Thiazide diuretics reduce blood volume by

enhancing the excretion of sodium and water, leading to a lowering of blood pressure. Studies have shown that thiazide diuretics significantly reduce the risk of cardiovascular events and stroke.

<u>Loop Diuretics</u>   Furosemide and Bumetanide are examples of loop diuretics. These are also primarily used in patients with heart failure or chronic kidney disease where excess fluid in the body is a concern. Loop diuretics act on a part of the filtering unit in the kidney called the loop of Henle causing an increase in urine output. They are more potent than thiazides but may cause electrolyte imbalances and require close monitoring. They are preferred in patients who have heart failure.

<u>Potassium-Sparing Diuretics</u>   Spironolactone, Eplerenone and Amiloride are examples of this group of diuretics. They are often combined with other diuretics to prevent the loss of potassium from the body. These diuretics permit the excretion of sodium and water while conserving potassium. Spironolactone is particularly useful in treating resistant HTN, a form of hypertension that does not respond to standard treatment. They cannot be used when kidney disease is present as it can cause excess retention of potassium leading to high blood levels of potassium (*hyperkalemia*).

Beta-Blockers

Beta-blockers are another class of drugs that help reduce blood pressure by lowering heart rate and reducing the workload on the heart. Beta-blockers are typically recommended for patients with conditions like *Angina* (chest pain of coronary artery disease), a history of heart attacks, or heart failure.

Selective Beta-Blockers   Exemplified by the medications Metoprolol, Bisoprolol, Nebivolol and Atenolol, these act on specific receptors in the heart. These receptors regulate the functions of the heart like heart rate and force with the heart contracts. Thus the beta blockers slow the heart rate and decrease output of blood from the heart, thereby reducing blood pressure. While not as effective as other drugs in lowering blood pressure, beta-blockers provide additional benefits for certain heart conditions. They are used in patients who have had a heart attack.

Non-Selective Beta-Blockers   These are used in conditions such as migraines and certain types of *Arrhythmias* (irregular heart beat). Propranolol, Labetalol, Sotalol, Carvedilol and Nadolol are examples of this type. They are termed 'non-selective' as they affect both the heart and blood vessels. However, they are not typically the first choice for treating HTN due to potential side effects, especially in patients with asthma.

ACE Inhibitors (Angiotensin-Converting Enzyme Inhibitors)

ACE inhibitors are a popular choice for managing HTN, particularly in patients with diabetes, chronic kidney disease, or heart failure. Exemplified by Lisinopril, Enalapril, Benazepril Captopril, Fosinopril, Perindopril, Quinapril, Ramipril, and Trandolapril, these medications act to *dilate* (widen) the blood vessels and reduce the production of *Aldosterone*, (an adrenal hormone) This results in a reduction in blood pressure.

ACE inhibitors have been proven to reduce the risk of cardiovascular events and slow down the progression of kidney disease. Patients who take ACE inhibitors need regular monitoring for potential side effects, such as *Hyperkalemia* (high potassium levels) and *Angioedema* (allergic swelling under the skin). Cough is a frequent troublesome side effect in about 15% of patients.

ARBs (Angiotensin II Receptor Blockers)

Angiotensin II receptor blockers (**ARBs**) are similar to ACE inhibitors and are often prescribed when patients experience side effects like cough with ACE inhibitors. The medications Losartan, Telmisartan, Valsartan, Candesartan, Irbesartan and Olmesartan belong to this group. They help to relax the blood vessels and lower blood pressure. ARBs provide similar blood pressure control and cardiovascular protection as ACE inhibitors but tend to be better tolerated as they seldom produce side effects like cough.

Calcium Channel Blockers

Calcium channel blockers prevent calcium from entering the cells of the heart and blood vessel walls, leading to the relaxation of blood vessels. Calcium is an important molecule which helps the contraction of the heart muscle. By blocking the entry of calcium into the cells of the blood vessels, the medication relaxes the smooth muscle in the arterial walls, which leads to *Vasodilation* (widening of blood vessel) and a reduction in blood pressure.

<u>Dihydropyridines</u> Amlodipine, Felodipine and Nifedipine belong to this group. They are particularly effective in older adults and those with *Isolated systolic hypertension.* [See Chapter 12 on *Isolated Systolic Hypertension*]. Calcium channel blockers have been shown to significantly lower the risk of stroke and heart attack in hypertensive patients.

However, they do have some side effects. Swelling of the ankles and feet is a common side effect, especially at higher doses.

<u>Non-Dihydropyridines</u>   These are used in patients who have both hypertension and arrhythmias or angina. Verapamil and Diltiazem belong to this category. In addition to relaxing the blood vessels, these medications also slow the heart rate, which can be beneficial for patients with certain heart conditions like *arrhythmias* (abnormal heart rhythm). These drugs thus are helpful in controlling the fast irregular heart rates of arrhythmias. However, they should be used cautiously in patients with heart failure.

Alpha-Blockers

Alpha-blockers are less commonly used for treating HTN but can be effective in certain cases, particularly in men with prostate problems. Doxazosin and Prazosin are the commonly used examples. They act by relaxing the blood vessels. These medications can effectively lower blood pressure, but they are generally not considered the first choice in treatment of HTN. Some patients may experience dizziness or lightheadedness, particularly when standing up too quickly (*Orthostatic Hypotension*).

Central Alpha Agonists

These medications work by targeting the brain's central nervous system to lower blood pressure. They are usually reserved for patients with resistant hypertension or when other treatments are contraindicated. Clonidine and Methyldopa belong to this group of medications. These drugs reduce the signals from the brain that increase heart rate and narrow blood vessels, thus lowering blood pressure. Side effects include sleepiness and, in some cases, rebound hypertension when the medication is stopped.

Direct Vasodilators

These are powerful drugs used in cases of severe or resistant hypertension. Hydralazine and Minoxidil belong to this category, and they work by directly relaxing the smooth muscle in the blood vessel walls, thereby *dilating* (widening) them and lowering blood pressure. Sodium nitroprusside is a direct vasodilator used in hypertensive crisis and has to be administered intravenously. They are very effective drugs but are usually used in combination with other drugs to avoid side effects like fast heart rate and fluid retention as they tend to increase the heart rate and retain fluid in the body.

Tailoring Treatment

Selecting the appropriate medication for managing hypertension requires a personalized approach. Physicians consider various factors to ensure the treatment is effective and safe for each patient. Here are some key considerations which the doctors use to choose a medication for the patient.

Age: Older adults may respond differently to certain medications compared to younger patients. Beta blockers may not be appropriate for the elderly as these patients already have a slower heart rate and beta blockers may further slowdown the heart rate.

Underlying health conditions: Diabetes, kidney disease, and heart problems influence medication choices. For example, a patient with chronic kidney disease cannot be given potassium-sparing diuretics.

<u>Severity of hypertension</u>: Whether to use one drug or a combination of drugs depends on how severe the hypertension is. When a patient has significantly high blood pressure, particularly when their systolic pressure is 20 mmHg or more above the target goal, or when they have a high cardiovascular risk and need a more aggressive approach to lowering blood pressure. In such cases the physician often prefers to initiate treatment with a two-drug combination instead of a single medication.

<u>Side effects</u>: Side effects also determine the choice of medication. Medications are chosen based on the patient's tolerance to minimize adverse effects. For example, some patients develop swelling of the feet with Amlodipine. Others develop cough when given ACE inhibitors. In them, an alternate medication has to be prescribed. Beta blockers may induce asthma in those prone to the condition.

<u>Ethnicity</u>: Certain medications work better in specific ethnic groups. E.g. Afro-Asian patients respond better to diuretics and Calcium Channel Blockers than white patients, while white patients respond better to ACE inhibitors and Beta-blockers. Combining diuretics with ACE inhibitors or Beta-blockers can be more effective than either medication alone for Afro-Asians.

Key Takeaways

- *Pharmacologic management of hypertension should be tailored to each patient based on their* medical history, comorbidities, and blood pressure targets.

- Common first-line medications include ACE inhibitors, ARBs, calcium channel blockers, and thiazide diuretics, often prescribed alone or in combination.
- For many patients, combination therapy may be more effective than a single medication in controlling blood pressure and reducing side effects.
- Regular monitoring of blood pressure and periodic adjustments of medications are crucial for achieving and maintaining optimal blood pressure control. Patient adherence to prescribed medication regimens is vital for long-term control and prevention of complications.
- It is important to educate patients about possible side effects of antihypertensive medications and adjust treatment as needed to enhance tolerability and compliance.
- RAAS inhibitors like ACE inhibitors and ARBs are especially beneficial for patients with conditions like heart failure, diabetes, or kidney disease.
- Medication choices may differ for specific populations, such as pregnant women, elderly individuals, and those with secondary hypertension or isolated systolic hypertension.
- Effective pharmacologic treatment of hypertension can significantly reduce the risk of cardiovascular events, stroke, and kidney disease.

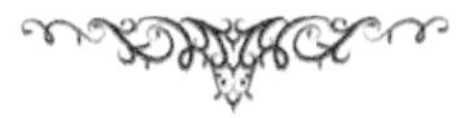

Chapter 9 - LABILE HYPERTENSION

Labile hypertension refers to unpredictable and fluctuating blood pressure levels, where readings may swing between normal and high. Unlike sustained hypertension, these changes often occur in response to factors like stress, anxiety, physical activity, or even emotional shifts. While it may seem less dangerous, labile hypertension can be challenging to manage and may eventually lead to more permanent high blood pressure if left untreated. Understanding its causes, symptoms, and treatment options is crucial for preventing long-term complications and maintaining heart health.

*Labile Hypertension is a condition where blood pressure (**BP**) levels vary widely, shifting between* *normal and elevated readings within a short period.* Unlike chronic persistent hypertension, where blood pressure is consistently high, labile hypertension involves episodic increase in BP, followed by periods of normalcy or even low readings. This unpredictable nature can make it more difficult to diagnose and manage.

Labile hypertension is usually identified through repeated blood pressure measurements showing significant fluctuation. For example, during an episode, systolic BP can rise above 140 mmHg, and diastolic BP may exceed 90 mmHg, followed by periods where BP returns to normal or lower levels.

Characteristics of Labile Hypertension:

Episodic Nature: The condition is marked by sudden, transient increases in blood pressure, often triggered by specific situations, like stress, physical activity, or environmental factors.

Asymptomatic Phases: Between episodes, the individuals may have completely normal blood pressure readings and may not exhibit any symptoms either.

White Coat Hypertension: Labile hypertension is often associated with "*White Coat Hypertension,*" where *the patient's blood pressure rises when he is in the doctor's office or hospital but remains normal at home or in other non-stressful environments.*

Potential for Progression: Labile hypertension can evolve into sustained hypertension if it is not diagnosed early and managed properly. This increases the risk of serious cardiovascular complications.

Distinction from Other Types of Hypertension:

Sustained Hypertension: *Sustained HTN is the condition where the BP is consistently high and does not fluctuate.*

Masked Hypertension: *Masked hypertension occurs when BP is normal in a clinical setting, as in the doctor's office, but elevated outside of it, making it harder to detect through routine checks.*

Causes and Triggers

Labile hypertension can be influenced by a wide variety of factors, including emotional, physical, and environmental triggers.

Psychological Factors

Stress and Anxiety: Emotional stress and anxiety are an important cause for labile hypertension. When stressed, the body releases hormones like adrenaline, which temporarily raise BP. Specific situations, such as exams, public speaking, or personal conflicts, can act as triggers.

Emotional Variability: Sudden shifts in emotions, such as anger, excitement, or fear, can cause spikes in BP.

Physical Factors

Physical Activity: Vigorous or sudden physical exertion can temporarily increase blood pressure. Individuals with labile hypertension may experience exaggerated increases in BP compared to those with stable BP.

Caffeine and Nicotine: Stimulants like caffeine (found in coffee, tea, and certain soft drinks) and nicotine (from cigarettes) can cause short-term increases in BP. These substances stimulate the nervous system, increasing heart rate and vascular resistance.

Temperature Changes: Abrupt changes in temperature, such as a sudden shift from a cold to a warm environment, can lead to temporary blood pressure fluctuations. When it is cold, the blood vessels *constrict* (narrow) to help the body retain heat. This increases blood pressure as more pressure is needed to force blood through the narrowed blood vessels. Conversely, in warm weather the blood pressure is usually lower because blood vessels *dilate* (widen), resulting in the body to cool down. In hot weather, excess sweating with subsequent loss of sodium may also lead to a fall in blood pressure.

Medical and Physiological Conditions:

Autonomic Nervous System Dysfunction: The autonomic nervous system regulates involuntary body functions such as breathing, heartbeat and intestinal movements, including BP. Any dysfunction in this system can lead to erratic BP control.

Endocrine Disorders: Hormonal imbalances from conditions like *Hyperthyroidism* (overactive thyroid) or *Pheochromocytoma* (a tumor in the adrenal gland) can lead to episodes of high BP due to sudden surges in hormone levels.

Sleep Apnea: *Apnea* means stopping breathing or low airflow. *Obstructive sleep apnea*, a condition where breathing stops intermittently during sleep, is linked to fluctuations in blood pressure. This happens because of oxygen deprivation and subsequent activation of the sympathetic nervous system, which raises BP.

Lifestyle Factors:

Dietary Salt Intake: Consuming a high amount of sodium can trigger temporary spikes in BP, especially in individuals who are salt-sensitive. Conversely, reducing salt intake suddenly may also cause BP to fluctuate.

Alcohol Consumption: Drinking alcohol can cause a temporary rise in blood pressure, followed by a potential drop as the body processes the alcohol. This is especially seen in binge drinkers.

Medications: Certain drugs, such as decongestants (used to relieve blocked nose), steroids, or stimulants, may cause temporary increases in blood pressure.

Managing Labile Hypertension

Managing labile hypertension requires a comprehensive approach that combines lifestyle modifications, pharmacologic treatments, and continuous monitoring.

Lifestyle Modifications: These have been discussed under the non-pharmacological management of HTN already. Hence, only a passing mention of these are made here.

- Stress Management

- Regular Physical Activity
- Dietary Adjustments - Reduced Sodium Intake - Limiting Caffeine and Alcohol
- Smoking Cessation

Pharmacologic Approaches:

<u>Antihypertensive Medications</u>: Managing labile hypertension with medication can be tricky due to the fluctuating nature of the condition. Low doses of antihypertensive drugs like beta-blockers, calcium channel blockers, or ACE inhibitors may be prescribed to stabilize BP. However, dosing and timing may need to be carefully adjusted based on the individual's BP patterns.

<u>Medication Timing</u>: Adjusting when and how often medications are taken can help align treatment with periods of high BP variability.

<u>Monitoring and Titration</u>: Continuous BP monitoring and close consultation with a healthcare provider are essential for adjusting medications to ensure they are working effectively.

Monitoring and Self-Management:

<u>Home BP Monitoring</u>: Regular monitoring of BP at home allows individuals to track their blood pressure throughout the day and identify any triggers for fluctuations. It is very important to use a validated BP monitor and follow proper techniques for accurate readings. [See Chapter 5 on *Blood Pressure Measurement*].

<u>Personalized Management Plans</u>: A tailored management plan should be created for each individual, considering their specific triggers, lifestyle, and health

status. This plan might include tracking BP trends, avoiding known triggers, and maintaining open communication with healthcare providers.

Behavioral and Cognitive Interventions:

Cognitive-Behavioral Therapy (CBT): CBT is a valuable tool for managing the anxiety and stress that can contribute to labile hypertension. It helps individuals develop coping strategies and manage emotions that could lead to BP spikes.

Biofeedback: Biofeedback is a technique that trains individuals to control physiological processes, such as heart rate and BP, through relaxation and mindfulness. This can help reduce BP variability.

Patient Education and Support:

Patients should be educated about what labile hypertension is, its triggers, and how to manage it. Understanding the condition reduces anxiety and promotes proactive management.

Joining support groups or participating in counseling can help individuals cope with the emotional toll of living with labile hypertension. Sharing experiences with others who have similar conditions can provide reassurance and encouragement.

Follow-up and Continuous Assessment:

Frequent follow-up visits with a physician are critical for monitoring the progression of labile hypertension. These visits allow for adjustments in medication and management strategies. Based on the data collected from home monitoring and feedback from the patient, physicians can tailor treatment to better manage the fluctuating nature of BP.

Labile hypertension is a complex and unpredictable condition, but with the right management strategies, it can be controlled. By making lifestyle changes, using medications appropriately, and monitoring BP regularly, individuals with labile hypertension can prevent the progression to more sustained forms of hypertension and reduce the risk of complications.

Key Takeaways

- *Labile Hypertension is characterized by sudden and significant variations in blood pressure, which can occur over minutes, hours, or days.*
- *Episodes of high blood pressure in labile hypertension are often triggered by factors such as stress, physical activity, caffeine, or emotional changes.*
- *Unlike sustained hypertension, labile hypertension is marked by alternating periods of normal and elevated blood pressure, making it harder to detect without regular monitoring.*
- *Key contributors include psychological factors like stress and anxiety, physical factors such as exercise and temperature changes, and lifestyle factors like diet, smoking, and alcohol intake.*
- *Management involves lifestyle changes, such as stress reduction, regular exercise, limiting sodium, caffeine, and alcohol, and quitting smoking.*

- *Pharmacological treatment may include low dose antihypertensive medications. But medication timing and close monitoring are crucial due to the fluctuating nature of the condition.*
- *Home blood pressure monitoring is essential for tracking patterns and identifying triggers, allowing for more personalized and effective management.*
- *Psychological interventions, including Cognitive Behavioral Therapy (CBT) and biofeedback, can help reduce stress and BP variability.*
- *Left untreated, labile hypertension may progress to sustained hypertension, increasing the risk of cardiovascular complications.*
- *Regular follow-ups and continuous adjustments to treatment are vital for managing labile hypertension and preventing its progression.*

Chapter 10 - SECONDARY HYPERTENSION

While most high blood pressure cases have no clear cause, known as primary hypertension, secondary hypertension is different. It arises from identifiable health conditions, such as kidney disease, hormone imbalances, or sleep disorders. Understanding and treating these underlying causes can often lead to better blood pressure control. In this chapter, we will explore the common causes of secondary hypertension, how it is diagnosed, and the treatment options that can help you manage and improve your condition.

High blood pressure, or hypertension, affects millions of people worldwide and is a major risk factor for heart disease, stroke, and kidney failure. While most cases of hypertension are categorized as *"Primary"* or

"Essential," where the exact cause is unknown, there is another type known as *Secondary Hypertension*. This type of hypertension occurs due to an identifiable underlying medical condition. We will explore the causes, diagnosis, and treatment options for secondary hypertension, offering practical insights into how managing the root cause can effectively control high blood pressure.

Causes of Secondary Hypertension

Secondary hypertension differs from primary hypertension because it has a direct cause, often related to another medical condition. Identifying and treating these causes can lead to better blood pressure control. Discussed below are the most common causes of secondary hypertension.

Endocrine Disorders

The endocrine system, which regulates hormones in the body, plays a significant role in hypertension. Several disorders of this system can lead to excessive hormone production, triggering high blood pressure.

<u>Primary Aldosteronism</u> (Conn's Syndrome)

This is a condition where the adrenal glands produce too much *Aldosterone*, a hormone that regulates sodium and potassium in the body. Excess aldosterone helps to retain more sodium in the body and lose potassium. The excess load of hormones thus causes the body to retain sodium, which increases blood volume, leading to higher blood pressure. The blood levels of potassium are very low in primary aldosteronism, and this can lead to severe muscular weakness, fatigue, abnormalities of the heart rhythm (*Arrhythmia*) and headache.

Primary Aldosteronism is more common in people with resistant hypertension—those whose blood pressure remains high despite taking multiple medications.

<u>Cushing's Syndrome</u>:

Cortisol is a hormone produced by the adrenal gland in the body. Cortisol is called the "stress hormone". When the body produces too much cortisol, it can lead to elevated blood pressure by increasing fluid retention and making the blood vessels more responsive to signals that *constrict* (narrow) them.

This syndrome often causes weight gain, particularly around the abdomen, a rounder face ('moon face'), a fat hump between the shoulders, sometimes called a 'buffalo hump', fragile skin that bruises easily and heals poorly and muscle weakness.

<u>Pheochromocytoma</u>:

This is again a rare tumor of the adrenal gland that causes excessive release of *Adrenaline* (*epinephrine*) and norepinephrine, hormones that raise both the heart rate and blood pressure.

Symptoms of Pheochromocytoma are episodes of heavy sweating, palpitations, and severe headaches often accompanied by high blood pressure.

<u>Thyroid Disorders</u>:

The thyroid gland situated in the front of the neck produced the hormone *Thyroxine*. This hormone regulates many body functions like how much energy the body uses, the heart function, brain development, bone health and many more vital functions. Both excess hormone and reduced levels of hormone cause the blood pressure to rise.

Hyperthyroidism: This is a condition when the thyroid gland becomes overactive causing an excess release of the hormone. This results in an increase in heart rate and cardiac output, resulting in an elevation of the systolic blood pressure.

Hypothyroidism: When the thyroid gland becomes underactive, the release of the hormone is reduced. This causes an increase in the diastolic blood pressure due to increased resistance in the blood vessels.

Kidney Disorders

The kidneys are crucial in regulating blood pressure. When they do not function properly, the body may retain too much sodium and fluid, causing an increase in the blood pressure.

Chronic Kidney Disease (**CKD**)

Hypertension and CKD are tightly linked; managing one often helps control the other.

When kidneys are damaged, they cannot filter out excess fluid effectively, leading to fluid retention. The damaged kidneys further release a set of hormones – Renin and Angiotensin which in turn constrict the blood vessels to raise the blood pressure. Chronic kidney disease is both a cause and a result of hypertension, creating a cycle where one condition exacerbates the other.

Maya, a 35-year-old homemaker, led a hectic life managing her household and caring for her three school-going children. Her husband, a busy executive at a leading pharmaceutical company, was often unavailable to help with family matters. Maya's days were consumed by cooking, preparing lunchboxes, and attending to the children's needs. Over the past few weeks, she began waking up with a persistent dull headache at the back of her head and neck. These headaches would fade after she took ibuprofen, so she dismissed them as stress related.

It was not until Maya confided in her close friend, Lissy, that she was urged to take her health more seriously. Lissy insisted Maya visit the local general practitioner, who, upon examination, discovered that her blood pressure was dangerously high at 176/116 mmHg. Alarmed, Maya's husband immediately took her to a well-known multispecialty hospital. After a thorough evaluation, Maya was diagnosed with Left Renal Artery Stenosis, a narrowing of the artery that supplies the left kidney, which can cause secondary hypertension.

She underwent angioplasty and stenting of the left renal artery to relieve the stenosis, and her blood pressure improved significantly. Although her symptoms resolved, she was prescribed a low-dose antihypertensive medication to ensure long-term control. This experience made Maya realize the importance of regular health check-ups and managing stress amidst her busy routine.

<u>Renal Artery Stenosis</u>

This condition occurs when the artery supplying the kidney become narrowed, reducing blood flow to the kidney. It can affect one or both renal arteries. This reduces the blood flow to the kidneys, which respond by releasing *Renin*, a hormone that raises blood pressure.

This condition can be caused by *Atherosclerosis*, a buildup of plaque in the arteries that is more common in older adults, or by *Fibromuscular Dysplasia*, a condition that tends to affect younger women and involves abnormal cell growth in the artery walls which tends to narrow down the inside of the artery.

Sleep-Related Disorders

Sleep disorders are an often-overlooked cause of secondary hypertension.

<u>Obstructive Sleep Apnea</u> (**OSA**)   OSA causes repeated episodes where breathing stops during sleep. This intermittent lack of oxygen activates the sympathetic nervous system, causing the blood pressure to increase.

Being overweight, male gender, or having a thick neck or narrowed airways can increase the likelihood of developing OSA. Snoring loudly, waking up gasping for air, and feeling excessively sleepy during the day are common signs.

Vascular Disorders

Vascular disorders are related to blood vessels. Some structural problems with the major blood vessels can also lead to secondary hypertension. Of these,

Coarctation of the Aorta is the most important. '*Coarctation*' means 'stricture' or 'narrowing'.

<u>Coarctation of the Aorta</u>

This *congenital* (present from birth) condition causes a narrowing of the aorta, the main artery arising from the left ventricle of the heart. The narrowing forces the heart to work harder, raising blood pressure above the constriction. The commonest site of coarctation is the part of the aorta situated in the chest. It often causes high blood pressure in the arms but weak or delayed pulses in the legs.

Medications and Substances

Certain medications and substances can also contribute to secondary hypertension.

Prescription Medications

<u>Oral Contraceptives</u>: Birth control pills containing estrogen can lead to fluid retention and increased blood pressure.

<u>Nonsteroidal Anti-inflammatory Drugs</u> (**NSAIDs**): Regular use of NSAIDs can cause fluid retention and reduce the effectiveness of blood pressure medications. Aspirin and Ibuprofen are examples of medications that can raise the BP.

<u>Corticosteroids</u>: Medications like *Prednisone* used to treat inflammation, can increase blood pressure by retaining sodium and excreting potassium.

Substance Abuse

<u>Cocaine and Amphetamines</u>: These drugs stimulate the sympathetic nervous system, leading to

dangerous spikes in blood pressure. The episodes of high BP caused can be severe and sometimes life-threatening.

Alcohol: While moderate alcohol consumption can have protective cardiovascular effects, excessive drinking can lead to high blood pressure, particularly with long-term use.

> *Andrew, an intelligent 8-year-old boy, had always been more fragile than his peers. Though eager to play, his physical limitations kept him from joining in the activities of his friends. His parents, hailing from a rural background, had assumed his frailty was part of his natural development and did not seek medical advice early on. When the family relocated to the city, they consulted a pediatrician, concerned about Andrew's apparent lack of physical stamina. During examination, the pediatrician noted a significant difference in blood pressure between Andrew's arms and legs. Further investigation revealed weak pulses in the lower limbs. Suspecting an underlying cardiac condition, the doctor ordered an ECG and Echocardiography, which confirmed the diagnosis of Coarctation of the Aorta.*
>
> *Andrew was promptly referred to a cardiovascular surgeon. He underwent surgery to correct the narrowed section of his aorta, and the procedure was successful. Postoperatively, Andrew recovered well. Within three months, he had regained his strength and returned to school, now able to participate fully in physical activities. His condition improved dramatically, and his blood pressure normalized.*

Genetic Disorders

Some forms of secondary hypertension can be traced back to inherited conditions.

Liddle Syndrome: This is rare genetic disorder that causes the kidneys to reabsorb too much sodium and lose potassium, thereby increasing blood pressure. It is an inherited disorder passed down in families.

Diagnosis of Secondary Hypertension

Accurate diagnosis of secondary hypertension is very important, as treating the underlying cause can often cure or significantly improve high blood pressure. The diagnostic process includes both clinical evaluation and advanced testing.

Clinical Evaluation

Secondary hypertension is suspected if the blood pressure remains uncontrolled despite treatment, or if it develops suddenly and severely at a young age. The physician suspects secondary hypertension under the following conditions.

- Onset before age 30 or after age 55.
- Severe or resistant hypertension.
- Hypertension is associated with clinical features that suggest an underlying condition (e.g., unexplained weight gain, muscle weakness, or episodes of sweating and palpitations).

History and Physical Examination

The physician suspects secondary causes for hypertensin if close relatives have conditions like early-onset hypertension. This could point to genetic causes.

The physician checks for signs like *abdominal bruits* (an abnormal sound produced when blood flows through the narrow renal artery.), swelling, or physical features associated with Cushing's syndrome or Thyroid disorders. A high blood pressure in the arms and a low blood pressure in the lower limbs suggests Coarctation of the Aorta. Many hormone disorders like hyperthyroidism and hypothyroidism have specific clinical features which lead the astute clinician to suspect these conditions.

Laboratory and Imaging Tests

These tests help pinpoint the underlying cause of secondary hypertension.

Blood Tests

Low potassium may suggest Primary Aldosteronism or Liddle's syndrome.

Thyroid Function Tests assess thyroid hormone levels and can help diagnose hypo- or hyperthyroidism, both of which can affect blood pressure.

Measuring and finding high hormone levels of aldosterone and low renin levels point to primary aldosteronism.

Testing the 24-Hour Urine sample for metabolic products of hormones Catecholamines and Metanephrines helps diagnose pheochromocytoma.

Elevated Cortisol levels in blood suggests Cushing's syndrome.

Imaging Studies

Renal Doppler Ultrasound or *CT Angiography* are tests that evaluate the blood flow to the kidneys and can detect renal artery stenosis.

Abdominal CT or *MRI* scans help identify adrenal tumors, such as those found in pheochromocytoma or Cushing's syndrome.

Echocardiogram is used to detect coarctation of the aorta. This test looks at the heart and the main arteries using ultrasound.

Specialized Tests

Additional advanced tests may be necessary in some cases. It is done in those cases where the laboratory diagnosis is not conclusive and also locate the side where the abnormality exists.

Adrenal Venous Blood Sampling is a test used to diagnose primary aldosteronism and determine whether the condition affects one or both adrenal glands.

Genetic Testing is done in rare cases to confirm a diagnosis of inherited conditions like Liddle syndrome.

Polysomnography (**PSG**) is a sleep study which may be conducted to diagnose obstructive sleep apnea. It is the gold standard for diagnosing OSA. The patient is monitored during sleep for episodes of apnea and other changes like changes in the brain waves, heart rate, blood oxygen levels, breathing, and eye and leg movements while the patient sleeps. This test which is the gold standard for diagnosing the condition and is done in a sleep laboratory.

Treatment Options

Treating secondary hypertension focuses on managing the underlying condition that is driving the high blood pressure. The targeted treatment based on underlying causes are described below.

Primary Aldosteronism

Medications like Spironolactone or Eplerenone block the effects of aldosterone and help control the high BP. In some cases, surgical removal of an adrenal gland is done to correct the condition.

Cushing's Syndrome

Surgically removing the tumor responsible for excess cortisol (either from the adrenal glands or the pituitary gland) can normalize blood pressure. Medications like *Ketoconazole* can lower cortisol levels when surgery is not an option.

Pheochromocytoma

Surgical removal of the tumor is the definitive treatment for this condition. Medications such as Alpha-blockers and beta-blockers are used to control blood pressure before surgery.

Renal Artery Stenosis

ACE inhibitors or ARBs are commonly used but must be monitored carefully. In selected patients, procedures like *Angioplasty* can open the narrowed artery. The term '*Angioplasty*' means using a balloon to stretch open a narrowed or blocked artery. Most modern angioplasty procedures also involve inserting a short wire mesh tube, called a *'Stent'*, into the artery during the procedure.

<u>Obstructive Sleep Apnea</u>

Lifestyle changes like losing weight and adjusting sleep positions can improve sleep apnea in many patients. *Continuous Positive Airway Pressure* (**CPAP**) is a machine that delivers constant airflow during sleep and can prevent blood pressure spikes during sleep.

<u>Coarctation of the Aorta</u>

Surgery is required to correct the narrowed section of the aorta. The treatment option depends on the severity of the narrowing, the patient's age, and other factors.

Surgery involves removing the narrowed section of the aorta and reconnecting the remaining ends. A patch may be used to widen the aorta. This procedure is more common for newborns and young children.

Balloon Angioplasty with Stenting is done more commonly in older children, teens, and adults. After treatment, patients will need lifelong follow-up care with a cardiologist to monitor for complications and re-coarctation.

<u>Thyroid Disorders</u>

Hyperthyroidism is treated with medications, radioactive iodine, or surgery. All of these can normalize thyroid function.

Hormone replacement therapy is the main treatment in Hypothyroidism. Thyroxine is available as tablets and the dose is adjusted to achieve optimal control.

<u>Chronic Kidney Disease</u>

Medications like ACE inhibitors can slow kidney damage in CKD. The specific condition which causes the kidney damage needs to be treated. Managing the specific kidney disease can improve blood pressure.

A multidisciplinary approach is needed in the management of secondary hypertension. It often requires a team approach, involving specialists such as Cardiologists, Nephrologists, and Endocrinologists, to treat the underlying condition.

After treating the cause of secondary hypertension, it is important to regularly monitor the patient's blood pressure and overall health.

Frequent blood pressure checks help assess the effectiveness of treatment. Periodic reassessment ensures the underlying condition does not recur. Even after treating the root cause, some patients may need ongoing medication to manage residual hypertension.

Secondary hypertension can be daunting, but the good news is that once the underlying cause is identified, it is often treatable. Whether the problem stems from hormone imbalances, kidney disease, or other health issues, addressing the root cause can significantly improve blood pressure control. By having a good understanding of secondary hypertension, the patient is one step closer to managing his condition and living a healthier life.

Key Takeaways

- *Secondary hypertension is due to an identifiable underlying condition, like endocrine disorders, kidney disease, or sleep apnea, and can often be treated by addressing the root cause.*
- *Endocrine disorders like primary aldosteronism, Cushing's syndrome, and thyroid imbalances are common contributors to secondary hypertension and can be managed through medications or surgery.*
- *Chronic kidney disease and renal artery stenosis frequently lead to secondary hypertension, requiring careful treatment to manage both blood pressure and kidney function.*
- *Obstructive sleep apnea (OSA) is a lesser-known cause of hypertension that can be effectively treated with lifestyle changes and CPAP therapy.*
- *Medications and substance abuse can elevate blood pressure, so reviewing your medication list and lifestyle choices is important in managing secondary hypertension.*
- *Diagnosis involves a combination of clinical evaluation, blood tests, and imaging studies to pinpoint the exact cause and guide treatment.*
- *Treatment focuses on addressing the underlying cause, with options ranging from medication adjustments to surgical interventions.*
- *Early detection and management of secondary hypertension are crucial for preventing long-term complications like heart disease, stroke, and kidney damage.*

Chapter 11 - HYPERTENSION IN PREGNANCY

Hypertension in pregnancy is a serious condition that can affect both the mother and baby, leading to complications like pre-eclampsia, eclampsia, and preterm birth. Managing high blood pressure during pregnancy is crucial to ensure a healthy outcome. This chapter will explore the different types of hypertensive disorders, their potential risks, symptoms to watch for, and the steps pregnant women can take to protect their health. Understanding and managing these conditions can lead to better outcomes for both mother and baby.

It has to be noted that HTN accounts for approximately 20% of all causes of mortality in women. Hypertension during pregnancy is a significant medical condition that affects both the mother and the baby. It is essential to be aware of the different types of hypertensive disorders that can occur during pregnancy, their associated risks, and how they are managed. Understanding these can help expectant mothers and their families take proactive steps in managing their health and ensuring a safe pregnancy.

Hypertensive disorders in pregnancy are classified into four main types: *Pre-eclampsia, Eclampsia, Gestational Hypertension,* and *Chronic Hypertension.* Each type presents unique challenges and risks, both for the mother and the baby. Let us look at these conditions in detail.

Normally, the blood pressure falls during the first 6 months of pregnancy. The maximum fall is within the first 6-8 weeks. It reaches the lowest point by 22 – 24 weeks and then may rise.

Pre-eclampsia

Pre-eclampsia· is a pregnancy-specific condition that usually develops after 20 weeks of gestation. *Preeclampsia is high blood pressure and signs of liver or kidney damage that occur in women after the 20th week of pregnancy.* It is marked by high blood pressure and protein in the urine (*proteinuria*), along with other potential symptoms. Preeclampsia occurs in about 4% of pregnancies.

Symptoms: Apart from high blood pressure, other symptoms can include *edema* (swelling), headaches, visual disturbances, and upper abdominal pain. Some women may experience sudden weight gain, difficulty breathing, or changes in liver function (as indicated by elevated liver enzymes). Low platelet counts causing bleeding and increased creatinine level in blood may occur.

Diagnosis: *A diagnosis of preeclampsia is made if the systolic blood pressure is 140 mm Hg or higher, or the diastolic blood pressure is 90 mm Hg or higher on two separate occasions.*

A urine protein measurement of 300 mg or more in a 24-hour urine collection indicates the presence of protein in the urine (*proteinuria*), a hallmark of pre-eclampsia.

Risk Factors: Pre-eclampsia is more common in the following groups of women.

- First pregnancy (Primigravida)
- Those carrying multiple babies (twins or more)
- Women with a history of pre-eclampsia during previous pregnancies
- Chronic hypertension
- Diabetes
- Pre-existing kidney disease
- Obesity
- Women over the age of 35 are at higher risk
- If the pregnant woman's mother had preeclampsia, the risk is higher

The underlying cause of pre-eclampsia involves abnormal development of the placenta, leading to poor blood flow to the placenta. This causes the release of certain toxic factors that damage blood vessel linings, leading to widespread inflammation, hypertension, and organ damage. This leads to preeclampsia.

Eclampsia

Eclampsia is the most severe form of pre-eclampsia, where the mother experiences seizures. It is *the new onset of seizures or coma in a pregnant woman with preeclampsia*. The seizures cannot be attributed to other causes, such as epilepsy.

<u>Symptoms</u>:   Along with high blood pressure and proteinuria, the woman may have seizures, which can be life-threatening to both the mother and the baby. Pain in upper right part of abdomen, severe headache with vision problems, confusion, breathlessness and unconsciousness are also symptoms of Eclampsia that may occur. Eclampsia can damage the liver, brain or kidneys and may be fatal.

<u>Diagnosis</u>:   Eclampsia is diagnosed based on the presence of seizures in a pregnant woman with pre-eclampsia. It is important to rule out other causes of seizures, such as epilepsy or a brain disorder.

<u>Management</u>:   Immediate medical intervention is required. The patient must be hospitalized in an intensive care unit. Treatment involves administering Magnesium Sulfate, which helps control seizures. The ultimate cure is the delivery of the baby, but the timing must balance both maternal and fetal risks. Delivery is the only definitive treatment for eclampsia, as it resolves the condition by removing the placenta which is the source of the problem.

Gestational Hypertension

Gestational hypertension refers to high blood pressure that develops after 20 weeks of pregnancy

<u>**without**</u> <u>the presence of protein in the urine or other</u> <u>signs of organ damage.</u>

<u>Definition</u>: Gestational hypertension is diagnosed when systolic blood pressure is 140 mm Hg or more, or diastolic blood pressure is 90 mm Hg or more on two separate occasions, but without proteinuria or other signs of pre-eclampsia.

> *Anita, a 26-year-old fashion designer, had recently married and was thrilled to discover she was pregnant six months later. Following her obstetrician's advice, she attended regular checkups and underwent routine tests. The urine did not show protein on repeated testing. Everything seemed normal until around the 24th week of pregnancy, when her blood pressure was found to be elevated at 146/96 mmHg. Concerned about the risks of Gestational hypertension, her obstetrician prescribed a low dose of methyldopa to control her blood pressure.*
>
> *Anita was also advised to adopt a healthy lifestyle, which included a nutritious diet rich in fruits and vegetables, with a reduced intake of salt and fat. Regular physical activity, such as light walking, was encouraged to help maintain her health during pregnancy. Fortunately, her blood pressure remained well-controlled, and she experienced no further complications.*
>
> *Anita's pregnancy progressed smoothly, and her delivery was uncomplicated. One month postpartum, her blood pressure had returned to normal, allowing her to stop the medication. Given her family history—her father was hypertensive—her obstetrician advised her to monitor her blood pressure annually and consult a physician for regular checkups to prevent future issues.*

Symptoms: Unlike pre-eclampsia, gestational hypertension does not cause protein in the urine or significant swelling. However, it requires careful monitoring because it can progress to pre-eclampsia.

Management: Blood pressure is monitored regularly, and only if necessary, medications are prescribed to control the blood pressure. Most cases resolve after the baby is born, but monitoring of blood pressure must be continued post-delivery. The goal of management is to maintain a safe pregnancy and prevent complications such as pre-eclampsia.

Chronic Hypertension in Pregnancy

Definition: *Chronic hypertension refers to high blood pressure that was present **before** the pregnancy or is diagnosed before 20 weeks of gestation.*

Management: Women with chronic hypertension need careful monitoring throughout pregnancy to prevent complications such as superimposed pre-eclampsia. Medications like Labetalol, Methyldopa, and Nifedipine are safe to use in pregnancy to manage blood pressure. *It is crucial to avoid medications like ACE inhibitors and ARBs, as they can harm the developing fetus*. If the pregnant woman is on these drugs, they are stopped before planning pregnancy and suitable substitutes given.

Risks for Mother and Baby

Hypertensive disorders in pregnancy can pose serious risks for both the mother and the baby if left untreated or poorly managed. Hence, understanding these risks helps highlight the importance of early detection and effective management to safeguard the health of both.

Risks to the Mother

Hypertension can damage the kidneys, liver, and blood cells. In severe cases, women may develop elevated *creatinine* (indicating kidney damage), liver enzyme abnormalities, and low platelet counts. Low platelet counts reflect problems with blood clotting and increased the risk of bleeding.

<u>Severe Complications</u>: Eclampsia is a dreaded complication of high blood pressure in pregnancy and the development of convulsions presages a serious complication. Pregnant women with hypertension are at higher risk of developing heart failure or even a heart attack. Elevated blood pressure increases the risk of stroke, which can have severe, long-lasting effects.

Placental abruption is a serious condition where the placenta detaches prematurely from the uterine wall, can cause heavy bleeding and threaten the baby's life.

Women with hypertensive disorders are at increased risk of excessive bleeding after delivery (*Postpartum Hemorrhage*) due to problems with blood clotting.

Risks to the Baby

<u>Intrauterine Growth Restriction</u> (**IUGR**): High blood pressure can reduce the flow of nutrients to the baby through the placenta, resulting in poor growth and

low birth weight. IUGR babies may require special care immediately after birth in a neonatal intensive care unit.

Preterm Birth: Preterm delivery may be necessary if the mother's condition worsens, leading to a premature baby who may face issues like respiratory distress and other complications like developmental challenges.

Stillbirth: In severe cases, especially in untreated or poorly managed pre-eclampsia, the baby may not survive and may be stillborn.

Neonatal Complications: Premature infants born to mothers with hypertension may experience jaundice, low blood sugar (*hypoglycemia*), or breathing difficulties after birth due to underdeveloped lungs.

Management and Treatment

Managing hypertension during pregnancy requires close monitoring and a comprehensive approach to protect both mother and baby. The US Preventive Services Task Force recommends low-dose aspirin 81 mg daily after 12 weeks of pregnancy for those at high risk of Preeclampsia. *But it is not given routinely to all pregnant women*. Calcium supplements also may prevent eclampsia. The recommended dose of calcium is 1000 mg per day.

Blood Pressure Monitoring: Managing hypertension during pregnancy involves a careful balance of monitoring, medication, and timely interventions to ensure the health and safety of both mother and baby. For women with mild hypertension, home monitoring may also be advised.

<u>Fetal Monitoring</u>:   Monitoring the well-being of the fetus is equally important. This is done through various methods:

- *Ultrasound (**USG**)*: Examination of the fetus using ultrasound provides images to assess fetal growth and development.

- *Non-Stress Tests* (**NST**): This test measures the baby's heart rate in response to movement, helping to ensure that the fetus is not under distress.

- *Biophysical Profiles* (**BPP**): Combines an ultrasound with an NST to evaluate the baby's health through a series of parameters, including heart rate patterns and fetal movements.

<u>Medications</u>

Antihypertensive Therapy: The   first-line medications for treating high blood pressure in pregnancy include Labetalol, Methyldopa, and Nifedipine, all of which are safe for both mother and baby. *It is important to avoid certain medications like ACE inhibitors and ARBs,* as they can cause birth defects or harm the baby's developing organs.

Magnesium Sulfate: In severe cases of pre-eclampsia or eclampsia, magnesium sulfate is given intravenously to prevent seizures and manage high blood pressure. The mother's magnesium levels are carefully monitored to avoid toxic effects of the medication.

<u>Delivery</u>

<u>Timing and Mode of Delivery</u>: For women with severe pre-eclampsia or eclampsia, delivery is the only cure. The timing of delivery depends on the severity of

the condition and how far along the pregnancy is. In severe cases, delivery may be required as early as 34 weeks. Induction of early labor is considered if the baby and mother are at risk.

Elective Delivery: In cases where hypertension is severe but controlled, doctors may recommend delivering the baby between 34 and 37 weeks to avoid complications. The decision depends on a careful balance of risks and benefits. The goal is to deliver the baby at a point where the risks of continued pregnancy outweigh the benefits.

Postpartum Care

Blood Pressure Monitoring: After delivery, blood pressure levels should be monitored for 6-12 weeks, as some women may continue to experience hypertension during this period. However, careful follow-up is necessary to ensure that blood pressure returns to normal and to manage any ongoing issues.

Continued Treatment: If blood pressure remains elevated after the postpartum period, additional evaluation may be needed, and long-term treatment may be required to manage chronic hypertension. Women with a history of pre-eclampsia or gestational hypertension should have long-term follow-up as they are at an increased risk for cardiovascular disease later in life. Regular check-ups help in early detection and management of any future health issues.

Patient Education and Support

It is important for women to recognize the warning signs of hypertension, understand the risks, and know when to seek help. This includes adhering to prescribed medications, monitoring symptoms, and attending regular medical appointments.

Managing a high-risk pregnancy can be emotionally and psychologically challenging. Access to support groups or counseling can provide valuable emotional support and help women navigate the stress and uncertainty associated with their condition. Support services can offer comfort and practical advice, contributing to better overall well-being during and after pregnancy.

Hypertension in pregnancy is a serious condition that requires careful management and monitoring. With early diagnosis, regular monitoring, and the right treatment, most women can successfully manage their blood pressure and deliver healthy babies. It is important to work closely with healthcare providers and follow their recommendations to ensure a safe pregnancy and delivery.

Key Takeaways

- *Hypertensive disorders in pregnancy include conditions like gestational hypertension, pre-eclampsia, and eclampsia, which can pose serious risks to both the mother and baby.*
- *Pre-eclampsia is a condition marked by HBP and protein in the urine after 20 weeks of pregnancy, and it can lead to life-threatening complications if untreated.*
- *Eclampsia is a severe form of pre-eclampsia, causing seizures, and requires urgent medical*

intervention, including delivery of the baby when feasible.

- *Gestational hypertension develops after 20 weeks of pregnancy, without protein in the urine, and usually resolves after childbirth but it can progress to pre-eclampsia.*
- *Chronic HTN is high blood pressure present before pregnancy or before 20 weeks of gestation, and it increases the risk of developing pre-eclampsia.*
- *Risks for the mother include organ damage, placental abruption, stroke, and heart failure, while fetal risks include preterm birth, intrauterine growth restriction, and stillbirth.*
- *Management of HTN in pregnancy involves regular blood pressure monitoring, fetal assessments, and the use of safe antihypertensive medications like labetalol and methyldopa.*
- *Magnesium sulfate is used in severe cases of pre-eclampsia and eclampsia to prevent seizures.*
- *Timely delivery is the only definitive treatment for pre-eclampsia and eclampsia. Delivery may be planned earlier if the condition worsens, or risks increase for the mother or baby.*
- *Postpartum monitoring is crucial, as some cases of hypertension may persist or recur.*
- *Patient education and support play a key role in managing hypertensive disorders in pregnancy, with close monitoring and adherence to medical advice essential for a healthy pregnancy.*

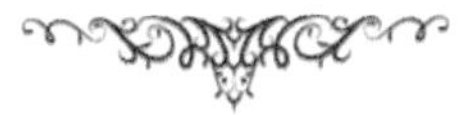

Chapter 12 - ISOLATED SYSTOLIC HYPERTENSION

Isolated Systolic Hypertension (ISH) is a condition where only the systolic blood pressure is elevated, while the diastolic pressure remains normal. This type of hypertension is particularly common in older adults and can signal underlying arterial stiffness due to aging. In this chapter, we will explore what ISH is, its causes, potential risks, and how it can be managed effectively. Understanding ISH is crucial for maintaining heart health and preventing serious complications.

Isolated Systolic Hypertension, commonly referred to as **ISH**, is a condition where only the systolic blood pressure is elevated, while the diastolic pressure remains normal. Specifically, a systolic pressure of 140 mm Hg or higher, paired with a diastolic pressure *under 90 mm Hg, is classified as ISH*. Unlike traditional hypertension, where both systolic and diastolic pressures are elevated, ISH is distinct in that it primarily affects the systolic component.

ISH is diagnosed after multiple blood pressure readings show that the systolic pressure remains elevated while the diastolic pressure stays within the normal range. Proper diagnosis often involves careful monitoring over time, since factors like stress or physical activity can temporarily raise blood pressure.

Prevalence

ISH is more common among older adults, particularly those over the age of 60. As people age, their arteries naturally lose elasticity and become like rigid tubes, making it more likely for systolic pressure to rise. Research suggests that 30-50% of older adults have ISH, making it a significant portion of the hypertensive population in this age group. According to a study by Whelton and others in 2022, ISH reflects a major aspect of hypertension in this age group. This highlights the importance of monitoring and managing blood pressure as people age. While it primarily affects seniors, ISH can also occur in younger people due to underlying conditions.

The development of ISH is closely linked to age-related changes in the arteries. Arterial stiffness is a major factor contributing to ISH. As we age, the arterial walls stiffen and lose their ability to expand and contract as efficiently as they once did. This stiffness forces the heart to pump harder to move blood through the body, leading to higher systolic pressure. At the same time, the diastolic pressure may not change as much, as the artery's ability to recoil and maintain diastolic pressure remains relatively stable. This phenomenon is largely why ISH becomes more prevalent with advancing age.

Causes and Risks

Aging: The primary driver of ISH is aging. As we get older, the natural elasticity of our arteries decreases, leading to increased pressure during the heart's contraction phase (*systole*). This loss of elasticity means that our arteries cannot expand and contract as effectively with each heartbeat.

Arterial Stiffness: Over time, arteries stiffen due to a variety of factors, including natural aging, the buildup of fatty deposits (*Atherosclerosis*), and other cardiovascular conditions. This stiffening is the key factor in the development of ISH.

Hyperthyroidism: Overactive thyroid function can also lead to higher systolic blood pressure. This condition speeds up metabolism, causing the heart to pump blood with more force.

Chronic Kidney Disease (**CKD**): The kidneys play a vital role in regulating blood pressure. When kidney function is impaired, the body may retain more salt and water, increasing blood pressure and contributing to the development of ISH.

Associated Risks

Cardiovascular Disease: Isolated Systolic Hypertension is not just a standalone condition. According to recent studies by Liu and others, in 2023, ISH significantly raises the risk of these cardiovascular events like stroke, heart attack, and heart failure. The heart works harder due to the elevated systolic pressure, which can weaken the heart over time leading to heart failure.

Cognitive Decline: Long-term studies have shown that high systolic pressure in older adults is linked to a greater risk of cognitive impairment and dementia. The strain that high systolic pressure places on the blood vessels can affect brain function, potentially leading to memory problems and other cognitive issues. Poor blood flow to the brain over time can lead to damage causing the cognitive decline.

Kidney Damage: Elevated systolic pressure can impair kidney function, worsening existing kidney issues or even leading to chronic kidney disease. Proper management of ISH is essential to prevent further kidney damage and maintain overall health.

Demographic Factors

Age: ISH is primarily seen in older adults, especially those over 60, as the prevalence increases sharply with age. It is a condition that becomes more common as people grow older, underscoring the need for regular blood pressure monitoring in senior populations.

'Old Age' or the 'Elderly' are defined as those above 65. Reason why they are special is that they may have the following features.

- More than one disease may be present
- Often take multiple meds
- May not get proper nutrition, especially if living alone
- Kidneys may not function well
- Increased risk of Stroke and Heart Attack

- Susceptible to lower blood pressure on standing – *Orthostatic Hypotension*
- Cognitive decline may be present – forget to take meds
- Many have ISH where SBP is over 140 but DBP less than 90

Pseudo hypertension or *Pseudo High blood pressure* is a condition named so and is caused due to calcification of wall of the arteries. Calcium is deposited along the arterial wall and BP reading can give falsely high values. No complications occur in these patients. Treatment does not alter the "high" BP. Other causes may be there for HTN like Renal artery stenosis. Kidney disease which have to be ruled out by appropriate investigations.

Gender and Ethnicity: Some studies suggest slight variations in ISH prevalence across gender and ethnic groups. For example, women, particularly post-menopausal women, may be at higher risk due to hormonal changes that affect the blood vessels. Certain ethnic groups may also be more genetically predisposed to ISH.

Treatment Approaches

Managing ISH involves a combination of lifestyle changes and, when necessary, medications. The goal of treatment is to lower systolic pressure without dropping diastolic pressure too much, as low diastolic pressure can also be harmful, especially to the heart.

Lifestyle Modifications

For many individuals, especially those with mild to moderate ISH, lifestyle changes can be an effective first step in managing the condition.

Diet: Adopting a heart-healthy diet can make a significant difference. One well-researched option is the DASH (Dietary Approaches to Stop Hypertension) diet, which emphasizes reducing sodium intake and increasing the consumption of fruits, vegetables, and whole grains. The DASH diet has been shown to lower systolic blood pressure in many individuals, especially when combined with other lifestyle changes. This has already been discussed previously. [See Chapter 16 on *Diet and Nutrition*].

Exercise: Regular physical activity, like walking, swimming, or cycling, helps improve cardiovascular health and lowers blood pressure. The American Heart Association recommends at least 150 minutes of moderate-intensity exercise per week for adults.

Weight Management: Achieving and maintaining a healthy weight is crucial for lowering systolic pressure. Even modest weight loss can lead to significant reductions in blood pressure.

Stress Reduction: Chronic stress can elevate blood pressure, so incorporating relaxation techniques such as meditation, deep breathing, or yoga can be beneficial.

Pharmacologic Treatment

When lifestyle modifications are not enough to control ISH, medications may be necessary. The treatment approach should be tailored to the individual, taking into account their overall health, the severity of ISH, and other associated conditions they may have.

Thiazide Diuretics are often the first-line treatment for ISH. They work by helping the kidneys remove excess sodium and water from the body, which reduces blood volume and, in turn, lowers blood pressure.

Calcium Channel Blockers like Nifedipine and Amlodipine are used to help relax and *dilate* (widen) blood vessels, making it easier for the heart to pump blood and reducing systolic pressure. They are especially effective in elderly patients with ISH.

Angiotensin-Converting Enzyme (**ACE**) Inhibitors and Angiotensin II Receptor Blockers (**ARBs**) are also used to help relax blood vessels and are often used in patients who have additional cardiovascular conditions, such as heart failure or chronic kidney disease.

Beta-Blockers are not typically the first choice for treating ISH but may be used in specific cases, especially if the patient also has a history of heart disease. They work by slowing the heart rate and reducing the force of contraction, which can lower systolic pressure. [See Chapter 8 on *Pharmacologic Management*].

In some cases, a combination of medications may be necessary to achieve optimal blood pressure control. This is particularly true in patients who do not respond well to a single medication or who have multiple cardiovascular risk factors.

In old age, the medications are typically started in small doses and the dose gradually stepped up in increments taking care to see that excessive fall of BP does not occur. Furthermore, the elderly patients should always have their BP checked after standing up for 2 – 3 minutes to avoid fall of BP on standing (*Orthostatic Hypotension*).

Monitoring and Follow-Up

Regular monitoring of blood pressure is essential in managing ISH. It is important to assess how well the treatment is working and make adjustments as needed. Blood pressure targets should be individualized, but most guidelines suggest aiming for a systolic pressure of less than 140 mm Hg in older adults. However, the goal should balance the risks of overtreatment, especially in frail elderly patients where too much reduction in blood pressure can lead to dizziness or falls. Hence the importance of checking the blood pressure while the patient stands.

Patients should be encouraged to monitor their blood pressure at home. Home monitoring provides valuable information for both the patient and healthcare provider, allowing for better management of the condition.

Patient Education and Self-Management

Educating patients about ISH is an important component of treatment. Patients who understand their condition are more likely to follow treatment plans and make necessary lifestyle changes. It is important for patients to know that ISH is a manageable condition. While it may sound alarming to have high systolic pressure, with proper treatment and lifestyle modifications, most people can control their blood pressure and reduce the risk of complications.

Taking medications as prescribed and attending follow-up appointments is key to preventing complications. Using a home blood pressure monitor allows patients to track their progress and detect any changes early, ensuring better long-term outcomes.

Isolated Systolic Hypertension is a common and serious condition, particularly among older adults. Left untreated, it can lead to life-threatening complications like heart disease, stroke, and kidney damage. However, with appropriate lifestyle changes and, if necessary, medication, ISH can be effectively managed. Regular monitoring, patient education, and adherence to treatment are essential to controlling systolic pressure and ensuring a better quality of life.

Key Takeaways

- *Isolated Systolic Hypertension (ISH) occurs when the systolic blood pressure is elevated ($\geq$140 mm Hg) while the diastolic pressure remains normal (<90 mm Hg), particularly common in older adults.*
- *Arterial stiffness due to aging is a major cause of ISH, reducing the elasticity of arteries and leading to increased systolic pressure.*
- *ISH increases the risk of serious health conditions, including heart disease, stroke, cognitive decline, and kidney damage.*
- *Effective management of ISH involves lifestyle changes such as a heart-healthy diet, regular exercise, and weight control, alongside medication when necessary.*
- *First-line medications include thiazide diuretics and calcium channel blockers, often requiring individualized treatment plans and frequent monitoring.*

- *Patients with ISH should aim to regularly monitor their blood pressure at home and attend consistent follow-up visits to ensure treatment is effective.*
- *Pseudo hypertension is a condition where falsely high systolic BP readings occur. This is due to thickening and calcification of the arterial walls seen in elderly patients.*

Chapter 13 - HYPERTENSIVE EMERGENCIES AND URGENCIES

Hypertensive emergencies and urgencies occur when blood pressure rises to dangerously high levels, typically above 180/120 mm Hg. In Hypertensive Emergencies, this severe elevation causes immediate damage to vital organs, such as the heart, brain, or kidneys, and requires immediate medical intervention. Hypertensive Urgencies, on the other hand, involve similar high blood pressure but without immediate organ damage, allowing for more gradual treatment. Understanding the difference between these conditions, recognizing symptoms, and knowing how to respond can be lifesaving. This chapter explains both conditions in simple terms and guides you on how they are treated.

High blood pressure may show no symptoms until it causes significant harm. But in some cases, hypertension can lead to critical situations known as *Hypertensive Emergencies* and *Hypertensive Urgencies*, which require immediate attention. We will explore these two conditions, explain their differences, recognize their symptoms, and discuss the treatment options available.

Hypertensive Emergencies

A *Hypertensive Emergency is a life-threatening condition in which blood pressure becomes severely elevated, typically above 180/120 mm Hg, and leads to acute damage to vital organs such as the brain, heart, kidneys, or blood vessels.* In these situations, the elevation in blood pressure can trigger events like a heart attack, stroke, or kidney failure. Immediate hospitalization is absolutely essential to avoid long-term damage or death.

The common signs of hypertensive emergencies include confusion, chest pain, difficulty breathing, and, in some cases, seizures or loss of vision. This happens because the blood vessels in these organs are overwhelmed by the sudden pressure surge, causing them to malfunction or, worse, rupture.

Signs and Symptoms

Hypertensive emergencies present with a variety of symptoms depending on which organ is being affected by the elevated blood pressure.

Neurological Symptoms: If the brain is impacted, symptoms can include severe headache, confusion, vision problems, or even seizures. These signs may indicate a condition known as *Hypertensive Encephalopathy*, where the high pressure causes swelling and dysfunction in the brain. It can also lead to a stroke, where a blood vessel in the brain is blocked or bursts. This is explained at length in the Chapter 15 on *Complications of Hypertension*.

Cardiovascular Symptoms: A person may experience intense chest pain, difficulty breathing, or irregular heartbeats, all of which can signal a heart attack or heart failure. *Acute Pulmonary Edema* is a condition where fluid rapidly accumulates in the lungs and the patient becomes extremely breathless. It is an emergency. In more severe cases, the pressure could cause an *Aortic Dissection* which is a tear in the large artery that carries blood from the heart to the rest of the body. This is a medical emergency. These are explained at length in the Chapter 15 on *Complications of Hypertension*.

Kidney Symptoms: High blood pressure can reduce kidney function, leading to decreased urine output or blood in the urine (*Hematuria*), both signs of acute kidney failure. This can happen because the kidneys' tiny blood vessels can be damaged by the pressure, leading to a loss of their filtering ability.

Immediate Treatment

Hypertensive emergencies require immediate and aggressive treatment to lower blood pressure and prevent further damage to the organs. The goal is to bring the pressure down rapidly but in a controlled manner to avoid causing additional harm, such as too sudden a drop in blood flow to the organs.

Immediate hospitalization, hence, is crucial for monitoring and treatment. Patients experiencing hypertensive emergencies are typically admitted to the intensive care unit (**ICU**) for close monitoring. Continuous blood pressure readings and evaluations of organ function are crucial to ensure the treatment is effective and safe.

In emergencies, blood pressure must be lowered quickly using intravenous (**IV**) medications. These include intravenous Labetalol, Nitroprusside and Nicardipine.

Labetalol blocks certain receptors in the heart and blood vessels, helping to relax blood vessels and lower blood pressure. Nitroprusside is a powerful drug that relaxes the walls of blood vessels, allowing them to widen and reduce the pressure within them. It works rapidly, making it suitable for crisis situations. Nicardipine is a calcium channel blocker that helps in relaxing the muscles of the heart and blood vessels thus effectively reducing blood pressure.

It is essential to continuously monitor blood pressure and adjust medications as needed. Rapid blood pressure reductions can sometimes cause low blood pressure (*Hypotension*), which is equally dangerous and can compromise blood flow to the organs.

John, a 40-year-old architect, had a family history of hypertension, as both of his parents were affected by it. Despite this, John had not undergone a proper medical checkup in over six years. Focused on his career, he often worked long hours, frequently overseeing construction projects. One afternoon, while supervising the development of a multistorey shopping complex, John suddenly felt severely breathless and experienced a tight, constricting sensation in his chest. Alarmed, his colleagues rushed him to the nearest hospital.

Upon arrival at the emergency department, his blood pressure was found to be critically high at 210/130 mmHg. Further evaluation revealed that John was in Pulmonary Edema, a life-threatening condition where his lungs were filling with fluid due to acute heart failure. He was immediately admitted to the ICU, where he received intravenous medications to rapidly lower his blood pressure and clear the fluid from his lungs. Oxygen therapy was administered via a mask to aid his breathing.

Over the next few hours, John's condition gradually stabilized. Within two days, he was transferred out of the ICU and eventually discharged on oral antihypertensive medications, with strict instructions to follow up regularly with his physician to manage his hypertension.

Hypertensive Urgencies

In contrast, a Hypertensive Urgency is defined as blood pressure levels that are equally high—again, usually above 180/120 mm Hg—but **without** the evidence of immediate or ongoing damage to vital organs. While serious, hypertensive urgencies do not carry the same immediate risks as emergencies. People with hypertensive urgencies may experience symptoms like headaches, nosebleeds, or shortness of breath, but they are not in immediate danger. Urgencies are treated more conservatively, often with oral medications to gradually lower blood pressure.

Signs and Symptoms

In hypertensive urgencies, the symptoms are less severe but still distressing.

A throbbing, persistent headache is common in hypertensive urgencies. Unlike regular headaches, these do not easily subside with usual painkillers. Difficulty in breathing may occur, though without the complications of lung or heart failure.

Frequent or severe nosebleeds (*Epistaxis*) can be a warning sign of dangerously high blood pressure. These nosebleeds can be frequent and difficult to control. Although these symptoms are concerning, the absence of organ damage means they can be treated in a less aggressive manner.

Immediate Treatment

For hypertensive urgencies, while the situation is serious, the treatment approach is less aggressive than for emergencies. The focus is on gradually lowering blood pressure over hours to days using oral medications. Oral medications commonly used are briefly mentioned below.

Clonidine is a drug that works by reducing the signals in the brain that tell blood vessels to narrow down, helping to lower blood pressure gradually.

Captopril is an ACE inhibitor that helps relax blood vessels, making it easier for the heart to pump blood. It acts quickly to bring down the blood pressure. Beta-blockers like metoprolol may also be prescribed to help slow the heart rate and reduce blood pressure. [See Chapter 8 on *Management of Hypertension – Pharmacologic Approaches*].

Alongside medication, patients are advised to make lifestyle changes to prevent future crises. This includes dietary changes like a low-sodium diet which can significantly help in controlling blood pressure. Processed foods, canned soups, and fast food are major sources of sodium that should be avoided.

Regular physical activity helps lower blood pressure by improving heart and blood vessel health. Maintaining a healthy weight reduces the strain on the heart and helps in controlling blood pressure levels.

The most important step after a hypertensive emergency or urgency is ensuring that the condition does not recur. Long-term management of hypertension is key to preventing future complications. Taking blood pressure medications as prescribed is essential. Skipping doses or stopping medication can lead to uncontrolled blood pressure and increase the risk of emergencies.

Regular check-ups with a doctor to monitor blood pressure and adjust medications if needed are crucial. Home blood pressure monitors can be used to keep track of readings between doctor visits. As mentioned, a balanced diet, regular exercise, and weight control are critical components of long-term blood pressure management. Reducing stress and limiting alcohol consumption can also contribute to healthier blood pressure levels.

Differentiating Emergencies from Urgencies

The key difference between hypertensive emergencies and urgencies lies in the presence or absence of end-organ damage. In an emergency, organs like the brain, heart, eyes or kidneys are already suffering from the effects of the high blood pressure. This demands immediate, intensive treatment, usually involving hospitalization and intravenous (**IV**) medications. Emergencies require swift medical intervention, often involving hospitalization and intensive treatment to prevent irreversible harm. The approach involves not just lowering the blood pressure but also addressing the acute damage to the organs.

In hypertensive urgencies, while the blood pressure is alarmingly high, there is no immediate risk to organs. Treatment can be managed more gradually with oral medications, and patients may not need to be hospitalized.

Hypertensive emergencies and urgencies are serious conditions that require immediate medical attention, but with the right knowledge and treatment plan, they can be effectively managed. Recognizing the symptoms and understanding the importance of prompt treatment can save lives. While hypertensive emergencies require hospitalization and IV medications, urgencies can be treated with oral medications and lifestyle adjustments. In either case, long-term management is the key to preventing future complications.

With some effort and commitment to managing blood pressure, many of the risks associated with hypertension can be avoided, allowing individuals to lead healthier, more fulfilling lives.

Key Takeaways

- *Hypertensive emergencies are life-threatening conditions in which severely elevated blood pressure (≥180/120 mm Hg) causes acute damage to vital organs, requiring immediate medical intervention.*
- *Hypertensive urgencies involve similar blood pressure levels but without organ damage, allowing for gradual treatment in an outpatient setting.*
- *Common signs of hypertensive emergencies include severe headache, chest pain, shortness of breath, and symptoms of organ dysfunction, such as decreased urine output or visual disturbances.*
- *Immediate hospitalization and the use of intravenous medications like labetalol, nitroprusside, or nicardipine are essential in managing hypertensive emergencies.*
- *Hypertensive urgencies can often be treated with oral medications like clonidine or captopril and require careful follow-up and lifestyle adjustments to prevent future crises.*
- *Monitoring and lifestyle changes—such as dietary improvements, regular physical activity,*

and stress management—are crucial to long-term blood pressure control and reducing risks.

- *The key difference between hypertensive emergencies and urgencies lies in the presence or absence of end-organ damage.*

Chapter 14 - HYPERTENSION IN CHILDREN AND ADOLESCENTS

Hypertension in children and adolescents is becoming an increasingly prevalent health concern, often linked to rising obesity rates and sedentary lifestyles. Once considered primarily an adult condition, high blood pressure now affects up to 5% of younger individuals worldwide. This chapter explores the causes, risk factors, and management of hypertension in youth, emphasizing the importance of early detection, lifestyle changes, and, when necessary, medical intervention. By understanding the impact of hypertension at a young age, we can take steps to prevent long-term complications and promote healthier futures.

Hypertension, or high blood pressure, is commonly associated with adults, yet it increasingly affects children and adolescents. Once rare, pediatric hypertension has become more prevalent in recent decades due to lifestyle changes, particularly the global rise in obesity and sedentary behavior. We shall discuss its causes, risk factors, diagnosis, and management. Understanding hypertension in children is crucial for preventing long-term health complications, including cardiovascular disease, which often begins with high blood pressure in childhood. By addressing this issue early, parents, healthcare providers, and communities can work together to ensure the health and well-being of the next generation.

Prevalence and Trends

Hypertension in children and adolescents, once considered a rare phenomenon, now affects 2-5% of this population worldwide, according to recent data (2022) by Lurbe and colleagues. This increase has been driven in part by the rising rates of childhood obesity. The modern lifestyle, which is marked by decreased physical activity and the consumption of calorie-dense, nutrient-poor foods, has fueled the spread of hypertension among the younger generation.

One in five children in developed countries are found to be overweight or obese. According to the CDC, 1 in 25 children aged 12 – 19 have high BP. Obesity is the main cause of HTN in children. *A child is said to be Overweight if the weight is more than 85% of children of same age and height (Percentile). A child is designated Obese if the weight is more than 95% of the kids of the same age and height.*

The prevalence of hypertension in children and adolescents is not uniform across the globe. Regional variations are evident, with industrialized countries like the United States, Europe, and parts of Asia showing higher prevalence rates compared to developing nations. This discrepancy is often attributed to differences in lifestyle, dietary habits, and access to healthcare. For instance, children in industrialized countries may experience higher rates of hypertension due to increased consumption of processed foods, higher levels of sedentary behavior, and greater overall exposure to risk factors. This is linked to urbanization, dietary patterns, and increased levels of stress in children from developed regions.

While measuring the blood pressure in a child, the width of BP cuff must be correct. If cuff is too large the BP reading obtained will be LOW   If is too small reading is HIGH. The rubber bladder of the cuff must cover 80% of the circumference of the arm. Different sizes of blood pressure cuffs are available for different ages and different arm sizes. The blood pressure of children of various ages is given below.

- Newborn BP   55/30 to 70/45 mmHg
- One month   70/40 to 95/60 mmHg
- 1 – 5 years   110/75 mmHg
- 6-12 years   120/75 mmHg
- Over 13 years   Normal BP Less than 120/80 mmHg.

Details can be obtained from the website given below.

(www.nhlbi.nih.gov/files/docs/guidelines/ child_tbl.pdf)

New born babies with low birth weight have HTN by adolescence. An overweight child can reduce BP by losing weight.

Risk Factors

Several factors contribute to the risk of hypertension in children and adolescents and understanding these can help in prevention and management.

Obesity: There is a strong association between body mass index (**BMI**) and blood pressure. Overweight and obese children are significantly more likely to develop hypertension compared to their peers with a healthy weight. Obesity is also linked to insulin resistance, which exacerbates the risk.

Family History: A genetic predisposition to hypertension exists, and children with one or both parents who have high blood pressure are at a much higher risk of developing the condition themselves.

Lifestyle Factors: Sedentary behaviors, such as excessive screen time and lack of physical activity, contribute to weight gain and increased blood pressure in children and adolescents.

Additionally, poor dietary habits, including high intake of salt and processed foods, exacerbate the risk. A lack of fruits and vegetables in the diet are also are key contributors to elevated blood pressure in youth.

Socioeconomic Status: Studies have shown that socioeconomic status also influences the risk of developing hypertension. Children from lower socioeconomic backgrounds often face challenges such as limited access to healthy foods, lower levels of physical activity, and higher stress levels, all of which can contribute to higher blood pressure.

The combination of these factors paints a clear picture: hypertension in children is often preventable with the right lifestyle modifications and early interventions.

Causes

As in adults, HTN in children is classified into two broad categories: Primary (essential) hypertension and Secondary hypertension.

Primary (Essential) Hypertension

In recent years, there has been a noticeable increase in primary hypertension in children, especially in adolescents. Primary hypertension occurs without a clear underlying cause, and it is closely associated with obesity and metabolic syndrome, much like in adults. The pathophysiology of primary hypertension involves multiple factors, including genetic susceptibility, environmental influences, and alterations in the autonomic nervous system. Over time, the sympathetic nervous system may become overactive, leading to increased heart rate and blood vessel constriction, contributing to the development of hypertension.

In addition, children with a family history of hypertension or cardiovascular disease are at a higher risk of developing primary hypertension themselves.

Factors such as diet, physical inactivity, and stress as has been discussed, also exacerbate this condition.

Secondary Hypertension

Secondary hypertension in children is more common than in adults and is often associated with identifiable medical conditions. The causes of secondary hypertension in children include:

Kidney Disorders: Conditions such as chronic kidney disease, *Glomerulonephritis*, a condition where the filtering units in the kidney become inflamed and damaged and *Polycystic Kidney disease*, where multiple cysts (sack like tissue filled with fluid) are present in the kidneys at birth are the leading causes of secondary hypertension in children. Kidney dysfunction affects the body's ability to regulate blood pressure, resulting in elevated levels.

Endocrine Disorders: Hormonal imbalances can lead to hypertension. Endocrine conditions like Hyperthyroidism, Cushing's syndrome, and Hyperaldosteronism are common such disorders. [See Chapter 10 on *Secondary Hypertension*].

Cardiovascular Disorders: Some children may be born with congenital heart defects, such as *Coarctation of the Aorta*, (narrowing of aorta) which restricts blood flow to the lower part of the body and leads to high blood pressure in the upper part of the body.

Medication-Induced Hypertension: Certain medications, such as Corticosteroids and Oral contraceptives, can cause secondary hypertension in adolescents.

Other causative Factors

Sleep Apnea: Obstructive sleep apnea, characterized by interrupted breathing during sleep, has been linked to secondary hypertension in children also as in adults. Untreated sleep apnea can lead to persistent high blood pressure and cardiovascular damage.

Genetic Syndromes: Certain rare genetic disorders, such as *Turner syndrome, Williams syndrome,* and *Neurofibromatosis,* are known to predispose children to hypertension.

Identifying the underlying cause of hypertension is essential for determining the appropriate treatment strategy, particularly for secondary hypertension, where addressing the root cause can often lead to resolution or improvement of the condition.

Management and Prevention

Managing hypertension in children and adolescents requires a comprehensive approach, with a focus on lifestyle modifications and, when necessary, pharmacological interventions. This comprehensive approach is essential to effectively control high blood pressure and reduce the risk of long-term health issues.

Lifestyle Modifications

Diet: A heart-healthy diet is critical for managing hypertension in children. The Dietary Approaches to Stop Hypertension (**DASH**) diet, which is rich in fruits, vegetables, whole grains, and low-fat dairy products while limiting sodium and processed foods, has been shown to effectively lower blood pressure. These have already been discussed. Salt consumption needs to be curtailed.

Physical Activity: Regular physical activity plays a vital role in reducing blood pressure. Children should aim for at least 60 minutes of moderate to vigorous activity every day, such as cycling, swimming, or playing sports.

Weight Management: For overweight or obese children, weight reduction through diet and exercise is crucial. Achieving a healthy weight significantly reduces the risk of hypertension and associated cardiovascular complications.

Stress: A variety of factors can cause stress in a child. This can include family issues like divorce or conflict, academic pressure at school, bullying, making new friends, major life changes like moving house, the death of a loved one, concerns about personal appearance, and exposure to traumatic events, all of which can contribute to feelings of anxiety and stress depending on the child's age and development level. These have to be adequately addressed.

Children should be encouraged to quit consuming caffeine containing beverages like coffee and colas. Smoking and vaping is not uncommon among adolescents and the use of illegal drugs is taboo.

Joy, a bright and active 16-year-old boy, excelled in academics and was known for his intelligence and diligence. However, his love for fast food and sugary soft drinks became a growing concern. An avid computer enthusiast, Joy spent much of his free time tinkering with his laptop or engrossed in video games. This sedentary lifestyle, combined with poor dietary habits, led to significant weight gain, making him overweight for his age and height. Both of Joy's parents, who worked in government service, had hypertension and were on treatment.

During a routine check-up, Joy's physician detected his blood pressure to be elevated at 150/104 mmHg. Concerned by this finding, the doctor ordered a series of investigations, all of which returned normal results. The diagnosis was clear: Joy's hypertension was largely due to his lifestyle. The physician strongly advised Joy to make immediate changes—reducing his intake of fast food and sugary drinks and incorporating at least an hour of physical activity into his daily routine.

With the support of his parents, Joy embraced a healthier lifestyle. Over time, he shed the extra pounds, and his blood pressure returned to normal levels. Though his condition improved, Joy was advised to maintain his new habits and monitor his blood pressure annually as a preventive measure.

Pharmacological Treatment

In cases where lifestyle changes are insufficient to control blood pressure, medications may be required.

The decision to start pharmacological treatment depends on the severity of hypertension and the presence of any underlying conditions or risk factors.

Common Medications: Antihypertensive drugs commonly used in children include angiotensin-converting enzyme (ACE) inhibitors, angiotensin II receptor blockers (ARBs), calcium channel blockers, and beta-blockers.

Monitoring: Children on medication require regular monitoring to ensure that the treatment is effective and to adjust dosages if necessary. Continuous follow-up is essential to prevent long-term damage to vital organs.

Prevention Strategies

Prevention is the key to reducing the burden of hypertension in children and adolescents. Early intervention, lifestyle education, and routine health monitoring can help prevent the development of high blood pressure.

Early Screening: Children at risk of hypertension, especially those with obesity or a family history, should undergo regular blood pressure screenings. Early detection allows for timely intervention, preventing the condition from worsening.

Health Education Programs: Implementing school-based programs that teach children about the importance of physical activity, healthy eating, and the risks of hypertension can empower them to make healthier choices.

Community Support: Community initiatives, such as family fitness programs and health awareness campaigns, provide essential resources and support for families in managing hypertension and promoting healthy habits.

Follow-Up and Long-Term Management

Long-term management of hypertension in children is essential for preventing future health complications.

Regular Check-Ups: Ongoing monitoring of blood pressure and general health is crucial to ensure effective management. Healthcare providers should schedule regular follow-ups to track the child's progress and adjust treatment plans as needed.

Transition to Adult Care: As children with hypertension grow older, they must transition to adult care. This requires careful planning to ensure continuity of treatment, particularly for those with persistent or secondary hypertension. By promoting healthy habits early in life and managing hypertension effectively, children can reduce the risk of cardiovascular disease and lead healthier, more fulfilling lives.

In conclusion, hypertension in children and adolescents is a growing concern that demands attention. With rising rates of obesity and sedentary lifestyles, it is essential for parents, healthcare providers, and communities to work together to prevent and manage high blood pressure in the younger generation. By making informed lifestyle choices and seeking timely medical care, we can safeguard the health of our children and reduce the long-term burden of cardiovascular disease.

Key Takeaways

- *Hypertension affects approximately 2-5% of children and adolescents globally, with rising prevalence linked to obesity.*
- *Key risk factors for hypertension in children include obesity, family history, poor dietary habits, sedentary lifestyle, and socioeconomic factors.*
- *Primary hypertension in children is often related to obesity and metabolic syndrome, while secondary hypertension is more common and linked to underlying conditions such as kidney disease, endocrine disorders, or cardiovascular issues.*
- *Management primarily involves lifestyle modifications such as adopting a heart-healthy diet, increasing physical activity, and managing weight.*
- *Pharmacological treatment is considered for children with persistent hypertension unresponsive to lifestyle changes, with medications like ACE inhibitors and ARBs commonly used.*
- *Early screening, education, and community support play critical roles in preventing hypertension and promoting long-term health in children and adolescents.*
- *Regular monitoring and planning the transition from pediatric to adult care are essential for those with chronic hypertension.*

Chapter 15 - COMPLICATIONS OF HYPERTENSION

High blood pressure, or hypertension, is often overlooked because it typically shows no symptoms. However, if left untreated, it can lead to serious health complications affecting vital organs such as the heart, brain, kidneys, eyes, and more. This chapter explores the dangerous consequences of uncontrolled hypertension, including heart attacks, strokes, kidney disease, and vision loss. Understanding these potential risks is essential to motivate patients to manage their blood pressure effectively and take control of their health.

High blood pressure, or hypertension (**HTN**), does not always have noticeable symptoms. However, left untreated or poorly controlled, it can lead to serious and even life-threatening complications. These complications affect various parts of the body, from the heart and brain to kidneys, eyes, and even mental health. Understanding these potential consequences is crucial for patients, caregivers, and anyone keen on managing hypertension effectively.

High blood pressure exerts excessive force on the walls of arteries, leading to their gradual damage. Over time, this wear and tear can contribute to a wide array of health problems, most notably within the *Cardiovascular* (heart and blood vessels) and *Cerebrovascular* (brain and blood vessels) systems, but also impacting other organs. We will explore the major complications of hypertension and their implications for long-term health.

Cardiovascular Complications

The cardiovascular system, which includes the heart and blood vessels, is one of the most vulnerable targets of hypertension. Hypertension-related complications develop gradually. The constant pressure of blood against the walls of arteries causes them to harden and thicken. This process, known as *Arteriosclerosis*, restricts blood flow and puts extra strain on the heart and other organs. HTN directly affects the heart and blood vessels. The heart must work harder to pump blood through stiffened, narrow arteries, and this constant pressure can lead to various cardiovascular issues. The coronary arteries which supply blood and nutrition to the heart are vulnerable to developing Atherosclerotic plaques and their blockage leads to heart attacks. (**See Fig 1**).

Heart Attack (Myocardial Infarction)

Atherosclerosis and Coronary Artery Disease Hypertension plays a major role in the development of *Atherosclerosis*, a condition where the arteries stiffen and become clogged with fatty deposits (*Plaque*). This can restrict blood flow and, when it affects the coronary arteries, leads to Coronary Artery disease (**CAD**). CAD not only increases the risk of heart attacks but also *Angina* (chest pain due to CAD) and *Arrhythmias* (irregular heartbeats). Atherosclerosis can also affect the other arteries in various parts of the body like the limbs, the arteries to the brain and the arteries in the abdomen. [**See Fig 2**]

One of the most well-known complications of high blood pressure is a heart attack. A heart attack occurs when the blood supply to a part of the heart muscle is blocked, usually by a blood clot in the coronary artery. High blood pressure is a major risk factor for heart attacks because it accelerates the process of *Atherosclerosis*—a condition where fatty deposits build up in the walls of the arteries. [**See Fig 2**]. These deposits, known as *plaques*, can rupture and cause a blood clot to form in the artery, blocking the flow of blood to the heart. This sudden blockage in these arteries can completely cut off the blood supply, resulting in the death of heart muscle tissue. Over time, hypertension accelerates the hardening of the arteries, making heart attacks more likely.

High blood pressure also makes the heart's muscle walls thicker and stiffer, a condition known as *Left Ventricular Hypertrophy* causing thickening of the muscle of the left ventricle. While this might sound like a good thing, it actually makes the heart less efficient at pumping blood, increasing the risk of a heart attack. Studies have shown that managing blood pressure effectively can significantly reduce the risk of having a heart attack.

A heart attack typically presents with chest pain or discomfort, often described as pressure, squeezing, or fullness. Other common symptoms include shortness of breath, nausea, sweating, lightheadedness, and pain radiating to the arms, neck, jaw, or back. Some people may feel only mild discomfort, while others experience severe pain. In a small percentage of people, a heart attack can occur without symptoms. A heart attack happens when the flow of blood to the heart is blocked, usually due to a buildup of plaque in the coronary arteries. These arteries are vital as they supply oxygen-rich blood to the heart muscle, and any blockage can cause serious damage to the heart.

When high BP is present combined with Diabetes, Smoking and Lack of exercise it increases a person's chances of having a heart attack by 15-20 times. A person with untreated HTN may live 10-20 years less than one without HBP. Control of high blood pressure lengthens the lifespan.

Prevention. Effective control of high blood pressure is crucial for preventing heart attacks and related complications in patients with hypertension. Following medical advice and taking prescribed medications are essential. Alongside, lifestyle measures such as maintaining a healthy diet, regular exercise, and avoiding tobacco are vital.

Two additional conditions, Dyslipidemia and Diabetes mellitus, must also be addressed to reduce cardiovascular risk. *Dyslipidemia*, characterized by high cholesterol and triglyceride levels, contributes to arterial plaque buildup, worsening hypertension and increasing heart attack risk. Regular lipid monitoring and treatment through diet, exercise, and medications like statins can help control cholesterol and improve heart health.

Similarly, managing *Diabetes* is critical, as high blood sugar damages blood vessels, worsening hypertension. Proper treatment with medications, such as metformin or insulin, along with lifestyle adjustments, helps control both blood pressure and glucose levels. This dual management significantly reduces the risk of heart attacks and other complications, improving overall cardiovascular outcomes for hypertensive patients.

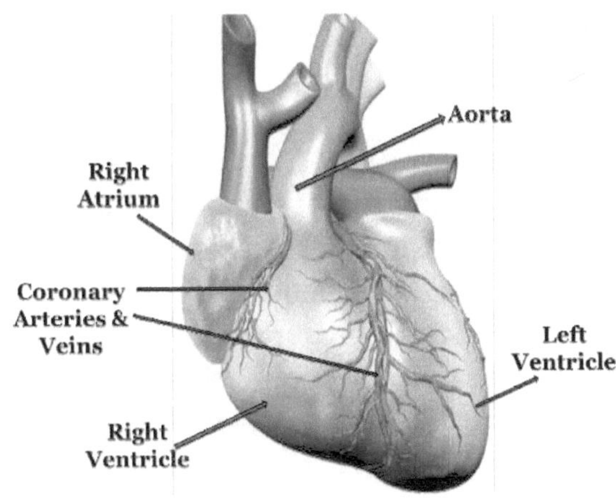

Fig 1 showing Coronary Arteries & Veins

Heart Failure

Heart failure is another serious consequence of long-standing high blood pressure. High blood pressure is the leading cause of heart failure because it puts an enormous strain on the heart.

Unlike a heart attack, which happens suddenly, heart failure develops gradually over time. As the heart struggles to pump blood against the increased resistance in the blood vessels, its muscles can weaken or thicken. The heart also enlarges. The heart becomes less efficient at its job, causing fluid to back up in the lungs, liver, or other parts of the body.

Symptoms include fatigue, breathlessness (especially when lying flat), and swelling in the legs or feet. These symptoms occur because the weakened heart is unable to circulate blood efficiently, causing fluid to build up in the lungs and other parts of the body. Although heart failure cannot be cured, managing blood pressure effectively can prevent further damage

Aneurysms

An *Aneurysm* is a dangerous condition in which a section of the blood vessel wall weakens and bulges outward, like a balloon. Hypertension increases the risk of aneurysms forming in major arteries such as the aorta. If an aneurysm ruptures, it can lead to life-threatening internal bleeding. Other common sites for aneurysms include the brain (*Cerebral aneurysms*), where they can lead to a stroke, and the legs (*Peripheral aneurysms*).

Regular check-ups to monitor blood pressure and imaging tests, especially in people at risk, can detect aneurysms before they become a major issue.

Arun, a 38-year-old software engineer, lived a fast-paced and stressful life, working long hours at a corporate job that required him to sit in front of a computer for 8 to 10 hours daily. With constant deadlines and frequent overtime, he had little time for family or recreation. His lifestyle led to significant weight gain, and his sleep suffered as he often managed with only five hours of sleep a night. The lack of exercise, poor diet, and chronic stress began to take their toll.

Over the past week, Arun noticed a tightness in his chest when climbing stairs or rushing to the office. He brushed off the symptoms as fatigue, but the warning signs grew more severe. One Monday morning, while enduring a heated conversation with his manager, Arun felt dizzy, broke into a cold sweat, and experienced intense chest pain. Moments later, he collapsed on the office floor.

Rushed to the hospital, Arun was diagnosed with an acute heart attack, and his blood pressure was dangerously high at 190/120 mmHg. An emergency angioplasty saved his life, but it was a stark wake-up call. The doctors advised lifestyle changes, a healthy diet, and regular exercise, along with medications for hypertension. Realizing the need for balance, Arun switched to a different company with a healthier work culture, allowing him to focus on his well-being and avoid future health crises.

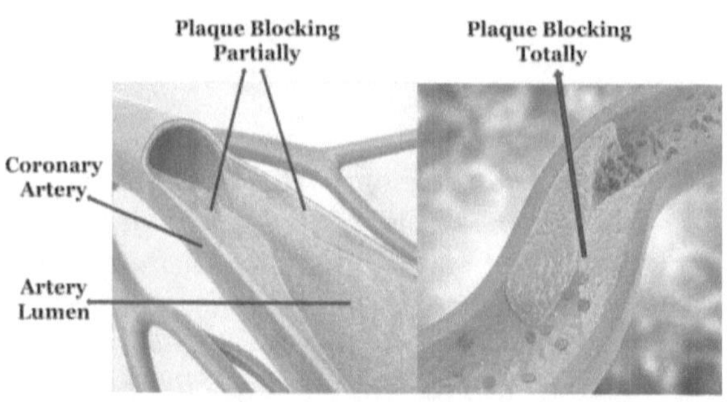

Fig 2 showing Plaques in Coronary Artery blocking lumen

Acute Pulmonary Edema

Acute pulmonary edema (**APE**) is a life-threatening complication which can occur in severe hypertension, where fluid rapidly accumulates in the lungs, making it difficult to breathe. This condition can develop suddenly and requires immediate medical attention to prevent serious complications or death. Essentially, the lungs become filled with fluid, preventing them from efficiently exchanging oxygen, leading to severe breathing difficulties.

Pulmonary edema can affect anyone, but it is particularly common in people with heart conditions, especially those with uncontrolled high blood pressure. Hypertension is a major contributor to this condition because of the stress it places on the heart and blood vessels, leading to fluid buildup in the lungs. While it can happen to anyone, older adults and people with chronic health issues like high blood pressure are more at risk.

Causes.   The most common cause of APE is a heart problem, especially when the heart is not able to pump blood efficiently. Very high blood pressure can thus lead to APE. High blood pressure puts extra strain on the heart, which can lead to fluid leaking into the lungs. In addition to heart-related causes, other factors like Infections (e.g., pneumonia), certain Medications, High Altitudes, Chest trauma, or exposure to Toxins can also lead to fluid accumulation in the lungs.

Pathophysiology. In a healthy body, the heart pumps blood effectively throughout the body. However, when high blood pressure remains uncontrolled, it overworks the heart, especially the left side. This increased strain weakens the heart, preventing it from efficiently pumping blood. As a result, pressure builds up in the blood vessels, causing fluid to leak into the air sacs of the lungs. This buildup of fluid interferes with normal breathing, causing a person to feel as if they are drowning.

Symptoms. APE typically causes sudden and severe symptoms, including, shortness of breath, especially when lying down or engaging in physical activity and a sensation of drowning or suffocating, which worsens when lying flat. A persistent cough that produces a thick, pink, frothy liquid, wheezing and a rapid, irregular heartbeat are also noticed. Dizziness, anxiety, and restlessness, often accompanied by a sense of impending doom and a cold, clammy skin and excessive sweating are often present. In APE, these symptoms develop suddenly and worsen over time.

Diagnosis. When someone is suspected of having APE, doctors perform a physical examination, focusing on the heart and lungs. A doctor will listen to your lungs for abnormal sounds like crackling or wheezing and check for signs like irregular heartbeats or low oxygen levels. Other clues, such as bluish skin and lips (due to lack of oxygen), increased breathing rate, and a very high blood pressure usually levels like 220/120 mmHg, help confirm the diagnosis. Further tests like chest X-rays, blood tests, and echocardiograms may be used to pinpoint the cause and severity of the condition.

Treatment. Acute pulmonary edema requires swift and aggressive treatment. The primary goal is to stabilize breathing and reduce the fluid buildup in the lungs. Common treatments include:

Oxygen therapy: Oxygen is delivered through a mask or nasal prongs to improve breathing.

Breathing support: In more severe cases, a machine may help blow air into the lungs to maintain proper oxygen levels.

Medications: Drugs that help the body get rid of excess fluid (*Diuretics*) are often used. If heart failure is the cause, medications may also be given to improve heart function. Most of the medications are given intravenously to ensure quick action.

Ventilation: In critical cases, a ventilator or respirator may be needed to assist with breathing.

For people whose pulmonary edema isn't caused by heart issues, treatments such as antibiotics (for infections) or steroids (to reduce inflammation) might be necessary.

Complications. If not treated promptly, acute pulmonary edema can lead to severe complications, including, damage to organs, respiratory failure, where the lungs can no longer provide sufficient oxygen, necessitating mechanical ventilation, heart failure, especially in cases where the condition is linked to uncontrolled high blood pressure or death, in severe and untreated cases.

Prevention.   Preventing pulmonary edema largely revolves around controlling its underlying causes, especially high blood pressure. Regularly monitoring and managing blood pressure through lifestyle changes, such as a healthy diet, regular exercise, and avoiding smoking, can significantly reduce the risk. In addition, taking prescribed medications for high BP and maintaining regular medical check-ups are crucial in preventing the condition from progressing. It is also important to avoid exposure to factors that may trigger fluid buildup in the lungs, like high altitudes or toxins.

Treating pulmonary edema focuses on earlier detection and advanced treatments to support heart function. Wearable technology that monitors heart rate and blood pressure in real time have been developed to provide early warnings for those at risk of heart-related complications. Additionally, new medications are being researched to help reduce fluid buildup more effectively and support heart function.

Acute pulmonary edema thus is a serious, life-threatening condition often linked to uncontrolled high blood pressure. Immediate treatment is essential, and proper management of hypertension can greatly reduce the risk of this condition.

Aortic Dissection

Aortic dissection (**AD**) is another life-threatening condition which may occur in severe hypertension where a tear develops in the inner layer of the aorta, the largest artery in the body. This tear causes blood to flow between the layers of the aortic wall, separating them, or *"dissecting"* the artery. If this dissection spreads and the blood breaks through the outer wall, it can lead to fatal internal bleeding.

Prevalence and Incidence. Aortic dissection is not a common condition, but when it occurs, it is extremely dangerous. It mostly affects older men, typically in their 60s and 70s. Women can also experience this condition, although it is less frequent.

Causes and Risk Factors. The most significant risk factor for aortic dissection is hypertension. Over time, high blood pressure weakens the aortic wall, making it prone to tearing.

Other factors that may contribute to aortic dissection include:

- Men are more susceptible than women.
- People over 60 are at higher risk.
- Cocaine use can cause sudden spikes in blood pressure and cause AD to occur.
- Though rare, aortic dissection can occur in otherwise healthy women during pregnancy.
- Intense physical strain, like lifting heavy weights, can dangerously raise blood pressure and precipitate AD in susceptible individuals.

Pathophysiology. The aorta has several layers of tissue. In an aortic dissection, high blood pressure or some other trigger creates a tear in the innermost layer. Blood then seeps through this tear and spreads between the layers of the artery wall. This can reduce blood flow to vital organs and lead to serious complications. If the blood exits through the outer wall of the aorta, it can cause severe bleeding, often resulting in death.

Symptoms. The symptoms of an aortic dissection are often similar to those of other heart-related conditions, which can make it difficult to diagnose quickly. Often the symptoms are mistaken for a heart attack. Common symptoms include:

- Severe, sudden chest pain that may feel like a heart attack.
- Tearing or stabbing pain that can move to the neck, back, or abdomen.
- Shortness of breath and difficulty breathing.
- Sudden fall of blood pressure, often leading to fainting or dizziness.
- Stroke-like symptoms, such as numbness or weakness on one side of the body.
- Symptoms like stroke, loss of vision and mental confusion may be noticed in some.

Diagnosis. Diagnosing aortic dissection can be challenging because the symptoms often mimic other conditions, like a heart attack. However, imaging tests, such as a CT scan or MRI, can provide clear pictures of the aorta and help doctors identify a dissection. Early diagnosis is critical, as the condition can rapidly become fatal.

Treatment. Aortic dissection is a medical emergency. Treatment needs to be prompt and includes:

Medications: Drugs like beta-blockers are often used to lower blood pressure and reduce the stress on the aorta.

Surgery: In many cases, surgery is required to repair the tear in the aorta. The surgeon may either remove the damaged section and replace it with a synthetic graft or insert a stent to support the artery. It is an emergency procedure.

In some cases, particularly if the dissection is small and stable, doctors may manage the condition with medication alone, but this is less common.

Complications. Without treatment, aortic dissection can lead to several serious complications, such as:

Aortic rupture: If the tear extends through the outer wall of the aorta, it can cause fatal bleeding.

Cardiac tamponade: Blood from the dissection can fill the space around the heart called the *pericardium* preventing it from functioning properly, which can cause sudden death.

Organ damage: Reduced blood flow can lead to damage in vital organs such as the kidneys, intestines, and brain, potentially causing kidney failure or stroke.

Prevention. Preventing aortic dissection primarily involves managing the underlying risk factors, especially high blood pressure. Some steps include:

Controlling hypertension is the key to reducing stress on the aortic walls and preventing AD. Since it can dangerously raise blood pressure, avoiding drugs like cocaine is crucial. Regular medical check-ups must be done in people with a family history of heart problems or aortic disease should have regular heart and vascular health evaluations. Regular BP checkups are also important. Maintaining a healthy lifestyle which includes avoiding smoking, engaging in moderate exercise, and maintaining a balanced diet goes a long way in preventing this condition.

Prognosis. The prognosis for aortic dissection depends on how quickly it is diagnosed and treated. If caught early, the survival rate can be as high as 85% with prompt surgical intervention. However, if left untreated, aortic dissection can be fatal within a matter of hours or days. Long-term survival often depends on careful management of blood pressure and other risk factors.

Medical advances have improved the survival rates for aortic dissection. One such development is the use of *Endovascular Stent Grafting*, a less invasive procedure compared to open surgery. This technique involves inserting a stent into the aorta through small incisions, reducing recovery time and complications.

Aortic dissection is thus a serious and potentially fatal condition, often caused by high blood pressure. Early recognition and treatment are essential for survival. By managing hypertension and adopting a heart-healthy lifestyle, many people can reduce their risk of experiencing this dangerous condition.

Cerebrovascular Complications

Hypertension also has a profound effect on the brain. It affects the blood vessels supplying the brain to cause Cerebrovascular complications. The high pressure on blood vessels in the brain can lead to both immediate and long-term complications. The impact of uncontrolled blood pressure on the brain can lead to severe and life-altering conditions, including strokes, transient ischemic attacks (**TIAs**), and vascular dementia.

Stroke

Strokes are one of the most serious cerebrovascular complications of hypertension. High blood pressure is the leading cause of both *Ischemic Strokes,* caused by a blockage in a blood vessel and *Hemorrhagic Strokes* caused by a burst blood vessel causing bleeding in or around the brain. Patients may have small *Aneurysms* (bulging of arterial wall) in the arteries of the brain called '*Berry Aneurysms'* as they resemble a small berry hanging from a vine. These berry aneurysms are highly vulnerable to rupture if the blood pressure increases to high levels. In both cases, the brain is deprived of blood and oxygen, leading to the death of brain cells.

When a clot blocks the blood flow to a part of the brain, the affected area is deprived of oxygen, leading to the death of brain cells and resulting in an ischemic stroke. This type of stroke is the most common, accounting for about 87% of all strokes according to a report of the American Heart Association (**AHA**) in 2022.

Constant pressure on the blood vessel walls can cause them to weaken and eventually rupture, leading to bleeding within the brain causing a *Hemorrhagic stroke.* This type of stroke is less common but often more severe, as the bleeding can cause increased pressure in the brain, leading to further damage. Both types of stroke can lead to severe disability or even death.

Sudden numbness, difficulty speaking, loss of balance, or a severe headache are the warning signs of an impending stroke. Prompt treatment within the first few

> *Ravi, a 55-year-old businessman, had been aware of his high blood pressure for several years but never followed a consistent treatment plan. He often dismissed his condition, attributing his occasional fatigue and headaches to the stresses of running his own business. One morning, as he was getting out of bed, Ravi suddenly felt a sharp weakness on the left side of his body. He collapsed, unable to move his left arm and leg, and had some difficulty speaking. His wife, alarmed by the sudden change, rushed him to the hospital.*
>
> *At the emergency room, Ravi was diagnosed with an ischemic stroke—a blockage of blood flow to a part of the brain. His blood pressure was recorded at 170/120 mmHg, significantly elevated. He was immediately admitted to the ICU, where his condition was stabilized with medications aimed at lowering his blood pressure and managing the stroke. Despite timely medical intervention, Ravi faced a long and difficult recovery.*
>
> *Following his ICU stay, Ravi was transferred to a rehabilitation center, where he spent months undergoing physical therapy to regain strength and coordination. While he made significant progress, he remained on antihypertensive medications and committed to lifestyle changes to prevent future complications. This experience taught him the consequences of neglecting hypertension management.*

hours of stroke symptoms can reduce the likelihood of long-term disability.

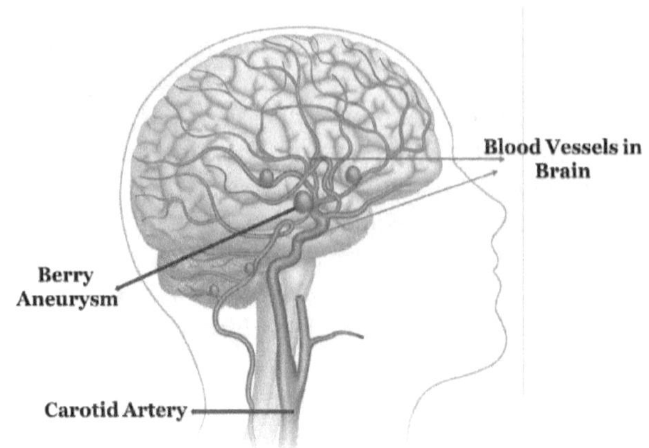

Fig 3 showing blood vessels to brain and a 'Berry' Aneurysm

Transient Ischemic Attacks

Commonly referred to as "mini strokes," *Transient Ischemic Attacks* (**TIA**s) are temporary blockages of blood flow to the brain. Although the symptoms usually resolve on their own within a few minutes to hours, TIAs should be treated as a serious warning sign that a full-blown stroke could be imminent. About one-third of people who experience a TIA eventually having a stroke, often within a year. TIAs cause similar symptoms to a stroke but may pass quickly. However, they should never be ignored.

Hypertensive Encephalopathy

Hypertensive encephalopathy (**HE**)is a condition where the brain stops functioning properly due to dangerously high blood pressure. It is a medical emergency that occurs when blood pressure rises so sharply that it begins to damage the brain, leading to confusion, severe headaches, and even seizures. Without quick treatment, this condition can result in coma or death, but the good news is that it is reversible if addressed promptly.

Prevalence and Incidence. Though hypertensive encephalopathy is a rare complication, it is still a significant concern in cases of high blood pressure emergencies. In the United States, high blood pressure emergencies make up less than 2% of all visits to the emergency room, but about 15% of those emergencies are due to hypertensive encephalopathy. It usually happens when blood pressure readings soar above 220/130 mmHg, although in some cases, it may occur with readings as low as 160/100 mmHg.

Causes. The primary cause of hypertensive encephalopathy is a sudden, extreme spike in blood pressure. Normally, the blood vessels in the brain can adjust to changes in blood pressure. However, when the increase is too sharp or too high, the brain's blood vessels cannot cope. This overwhelms the brain's natural defenses, causing fluid to leak into the brain tissue, which results in swelling and impaired brain function and leads to the condition. This is what causes the symptoms like confusion, headaches, and vision problems.

Pathophysiology. To explain it simply, the brain needs a constant, controlled flow of blood. When the blood pressure rises suddenly and dramatically, the blood vessels in the brain can no longer regulate this flow. The blood-brain barrier, which normally protects the brain from harmful substances, gets disrupted, allowing fluid to leak into the brain. This fluid buildup, called *Cerebral Edema*, causes the brain to swell, leading to dysfunction. It is like a water pipe bursting, with the pressure causing water to flood the area.

Symptoms.   The symptoms usually begin with severe headaches, nausea, and vomiting. As the condition progresses, it begins to affect brain function, causing confusion, personality changes, and irritability. Vision problems such as blurry vision or loss of sight may occur. In severe cases, seizures, loss of consciousness, and even coma can follow. If left untreated, the condition can cause irreversible damage, leading to permanent brain injury or death.

Diagnosis.   A doctor diagnoses HE by considering the person's blood pressure reading along with their symptoms. If someone with a very high blood pressure reading, typically over 220/130 mmHg, shows the symptoms already described, doctors may suspect hypertensive encephalopathy. Diagnostic tests may include brain imaging to check for swelling, blood tests to assess organ function, and an eye exam using ophthalmoscopy, which might show retinal changes like swelling and bleeding.

Treatment.   Treating HE requires immediate action to lower blood pressure in a controlled way. The goal is to reduce the pressure enough to relieve brain swelling without lowering it too quickly, which could cause other complications. Doctors use fast-acting medications like Nicardipine, Labetalol, Hydralazine, Fenoldopam, and Sodium Nitroprusside to gradually bring blood pressure down to safer levels. These medications work quickly and are usually given in a hospital setting to allow close monitoring. Most people begin to recover once their blood pressure is under control, though it may take a few days to weeks to fully feel better.

Complications. If not treated promptly, HE can lead to several severe complications. These include permanent brain damage due to swelling, bleeding in the brain (*hemorrhage*), or even stroke. Other organs may also be affected, causing kidney failure, heart attacks, or damage to the retina, which can cause vision loss. In the worst-case scenario, the condition can progress to coma and death. Even with treatment, up to 50% of people with hypertensive emergencies may die within six months if they do not receive proper care.

Prevention. The best way to prevent hypertensive encephalopathy is to manage high blood pressure effectively. Regular checkups, medication, and lifestyle changes can keep blood pressure under control. If you have high blood pressure, it is essential to take your medications as prescribed and avoid missing doses. Regular monitoring is necessary to catch dangerous spikes early before they lead to more serious problems.

While treatment approaches for HE have not changed drastically in recent years, advancements in fast-acting blood pressure medications have improved patient outcomes. There is also growing awareness of the importance of personalized treatment plans that consider an individual's specific health profile, which can reduce complications.

Hypertensive encephalopathy serves as a stark reminder of how important it is to control high blood pressure. It is a condition that can escalate quickly but is preventable and treatable if managed early. Awareness, regular blood pressure monitoring, and quick medical intervention are key to reducing the risks associated with this life-threatening condition.

Vascular Dementia

The word *dementia* means decline in brain function. *Vascular Dementia* is a type of dementia caused by reduced blood flow to the brain, leading to damage to the brain's white matter and the death of brain cells. This condition is often linked to a history of strokes or other conditions that affect the blood vessels in the brain, including hypertension.

Over time, hypertension can damage the blood vessels in the brain, leading to vascular dementia. This condition occurs when reduced blood flow harms the brain's ability to function, causing issues with memory, thinking, and reasoning.

Difficulty concentrating, forgetfulness, and confusion are common. This condition is often progressive but can be managed by controlling blood pressure and making lifestyle changes. Unlike other forms of dementia, such as Alzheimer's disease, the symptoms of vascular dementia can occur suddenly, particularly after a stroke or TIA. However, in many cases, the cognitive decline is gradual, as the damage accumulates over time.

Renal (Kidney) Complications

Hypertension can have serious repercussions for the kidneys. The kidneys play a vital role in filtering waste from the blood, and they depend on healthy blood vessels to function properly. High blood pressure can damage the arteries around the kidneys, leading to a condition called *Chronic Kidney Disease* (**CKD**). This occurs when the kidneys lose their ability to filter waste effectively.

Chronic Kidney Disease

Chronic Kidney Disease is a progressive condition where the kidneys gradually lose their ability to function properly over time. Persistent hypertension exerts excessive pressure on the blood vessels within the kidneys. Over time, this increased pressure can cause the tiny blood vessels (*Glomeruli*) in the kidneys to become damaged.

The damage impairs the kidneys' ability to filter waste and regulate fluid balance effectively. This results in waste and excess fluids to accumulate in the body. Left untreated, CKD can progress to kidney failure, requiring dialysis or a kidney transplant.

Symptoms of CKD. CKD often develops slowly, with few noticeable symptoms in the early stages. But as kidney function declines, patients may experience fatigue, swelling in the legs, and changes in urination patterns.

End-Stage Renal Disease (**ESRD**) is the final, severe stage of chronic kidney disease, where the kidneys are functioning at less than 10% of their normal capacity. At this stage, the kidneys can no longer adequately filter waste from the blood, leading to life-threatening complications. The progression from CKD to ESRD involves severe damage to the kidneys, often due to prolonged high blood pressure. This stage of kidney failure requires intensive medical intervention to sustain life. Treatment options for ESRD include *dialysis*, a procedure that artificially removes waste and excess fluids from the blood using a dialysis machine, or a kidney transplant, where a healthy kidney from a donor is surgically implanted into the patient with ESRD.

Monitoring kidney function through tests like serum creatinine levels and estimated glomerular filtration rate (eGFR) can help in early diagnosis and management. Managing blood pressure, staying hydrated, and maintaining a healthy diet can slow the progression of CKD.

Eye (Ocular) Complications

Hypertension does not just affect major organs—it can also impact vision. *Hypertensive Retinopathy* occurs when high blood pressure causes damage to the blood vessels in the retina, the light-sensitive layer at the back of the eye. It is the part of the eye responsible for capturing visual images. The blood vessels in the eyes are delicate and can be adversely affected by sustained high blood pressure, leading to several ocular complications.

Hypertensive Retinopathy

Severe and uncontrolled HTN can damage the delicate blood vessels in the retina. The retina is the layer of tissue lining the back of the eye. When light falls on the retina, they are converted into nerve signals that are sent to the brain through the optic nerve. Damage to the retina from high blood pressure is called *Hypertensive Retinopathy* (**HR**). Hypertensive retinopathy is usually asymptomatic until the changes are advanced. The damage to the retinal arteries once occurred cannot be reversed. The *Optic Disc*, also called the *Optic Nerve Head*, is a round whitish section at the back of the eye. It is the portion where the optic nerve connects with the retina. The retina's main arteries and veins enter the eye at the optic disc. The *Macula* is an oval-shaped spot in the center of the retina that is responsible for central vision, color vision, and fine details.

Chronic HTN puts extra pressure on the blood vessels in the retina, leading to changes such as thickening of the vessel walls, narrowing of the vessels, and leakage of fluid. These changes can cause bleeding, swelling, and damage to the retina. Damage to the blood vessels in the retina can lead to blurred vision, vision loss, or even blindness if left untreated. People with high blood pressure are at a greater risk, especially if they also have diabetes.

The following are the changes occurring in the retina in HR:

- Bleeding in the retina that appears as a dot, a blot or shaped like a 'flame'. These are called *Retinal hemorrhages*.
- Fatty deposits in the retina appear (*Retinal exudates*) and are also known as 'Cotton Wool' spots.
- Narrowing of the tiny blood vessels in the retina (*Arteriolar constriction*) is also seen.

- The walls of the tiny blood vessels in the retina thicken.
- Swelling of the optic disc occurs in late stages of HR and is known as *Papilledema.*
- Tiny red dots in the retina are seen closely related to the tiny blood vessels. These are small bulging in the wall of the retinal arteries and are called *Microaneurysms.*
- Changes may appear in the lining of the retina and gives a moth-eaten appearance.

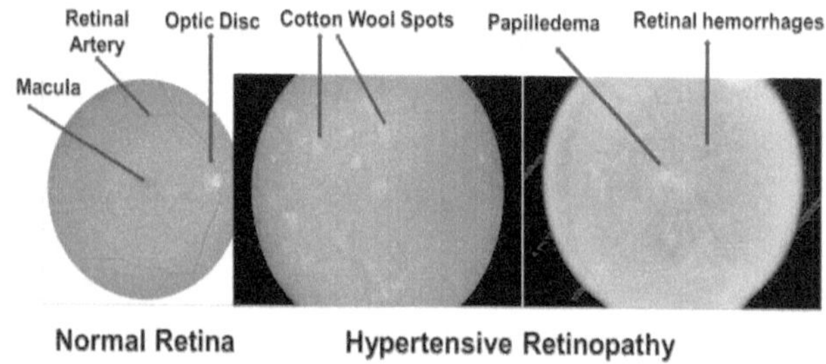

Fig 4. Showing Normal Retina and Hypertensive Retinopathy

Symptoms of hypertensive retinopathy include eye pain, blurred vision, and sudden vision loss. Early detection through regular eye exams is key to preventing permanent damage.

Glaucoma

Glaucoma is a group of eye conditions characterized by increased pressure within the eyeball, which can damage the optic nerve. Elevated blood pressure can influence eye pressure by affecting the blood flow to the optic nerve and the drainage of the fluid inside the eye (*Aqueous Humor*). This increased pressure can lead to damage of the optic nerve fibers, causing vision loss and, if untreated, potentially leading to blindness. Glaucoma is often asymptomatic in its early stages.

Untreated hypertension can lead to severe vision loss, including potential blindness, due to the cumulative effects of hypertensive retinopathy and glaucoma. Patients with hypertension should have routine eye exams to detect early signs of retinopathy and glaucoma.

Peripheral Artery Disease

Peripheral Artery Disease (**PAD**) is a common condition that affects the arteries supplying blood to the limbs, primarily the legs. Hypertension can also affect the arteries outside the heart and brain. Peripheral artery disease (PAD) is a condition where narrowed arteries reduce blood flow to the limbs, usually the legs. This can cause pain in the muscles when walking, known as *claudication*, and increases the risk of infections and ulcers.

In addition to pain, people with PAD may experience numbness or tingling in their legs and feet. The skin on the legs may also appear pale, bluish, or shiny, and wounds or sores may develop that are slow to heal. The reduced blood flow increases the risk of infections and, in severe cases, can lead to gangrene, a serious condition where tissue dies due to lack of blood supply.

As PAD progresses, the reduced blood flow can lead to significant complications, including pain and weakness in the legs, particularly during physical activities. The decreased circulation also makes it harder for wounds or infections in the legs to heal, increasing the risk of serious complications.

Smoking cessation, exercise, and medication to control blood pressure and cholesterol can help reduce symptoms and prevent progression. Medications may be prescribed to help manage PAD and associated hypertension. These can include medications to lower blood pressure as well as medications to reduce blood clots and improve blood flow, such as *Aspirin* or *Clopidogrel*. In some cases, more advanced treatments may be needed, such as angioplasty or surgery to open blocked arteries and improve blood flow. These interventions can help alleviate symptoms and improve quality of life for those with severe PAD.

Sexual Dysfunction.

Hypertension can interfere with normal blood flow, which can lead to *Erectile Dysfunction* (**ED**) in men and sexual dysfunction in women. Poor blood flow makes it difficult for the body to respond to sexual stimuli.

Healthy blood pressure management, exercise, and open discussions with a healthcare provider can help improve sexual health.

The complications of hypertension are far-reaching, but the good news is that most of these conditions can be prevented or managed by controlling blood pressure effectively. Simple steps like maintaining a balanced diet, exercising regularly, quitting smoking, and adhering to prescribed medications can make a significant difference in reducing risks.

It is important to remember that early detection and intervention are key. By managing blood pressure, people can live long, healthy lives, free from the serious complications that hypertension can bring.

Key Takeaways

- *Hypertension is a "Silent Killer": It often has no symptoms but can lead to serious, life-threatening complications if left untreated.*
- *High blood pressure can cause heart attacks, heart failure, atherosclerosis, acute pulmonary edema, aortic dissection and aneurysms due to the strain on the cardiovascular system.*
- *Hypertension is the leading cause of strokes, mini strokes (**TIAs**), and can lead to long-term cognitive decline like vascular dementia.*
- *It can also cause Hypertensive Encephalopathy, a dangerous complication if not promptly treated.*
- *Chronic kidney disease (**CKD**) often results from untreated hypertension, leading to kidney failure if not addressed.*
- *High blood pressure can damage the retina, leading to hypertensive retinopathy and glaucoma, both causing potential vision loss.*
- *Narrowed arteries due to hypertension can cause pain and complications in the limbs, particularly the legs.*

- *Hypertension can impact blood flow to the sexual organs, leading to sexual dysfunction in both men and women.*
- *Effective management of blood pressure through a healthy lifestyle, regular monitoring, and medication can prevent or mitigate these complications.*

Chapter 16 - DIET AND NUTRITION IN HYPERTENSION

In this chapter we explore how making informed dietary choices can significantly impact blood pressure levels and overall cardiovascular health. By focusing on a balanced diet rich in essential nutrients, adopting the DASH diet, and reducing sodium intake, individuals can effectively manage and prevent hypertension. This chapter provides practical advice on how to integrate these dietary principles into daily life, offering a pathway to better health through mindful eating and nutrition.

High blood pressure, or hypertension, is a serious health concern that affects millions globally. One of the most effective and accessible ways to manage and prevent hypertension is through diet and nutrition. Let us explore how a well-balanced diet can significantly lower blood pressure, with a focus on specific nutrients, evidence-based dietary approaches like the DASH diet, and practical tips for reducing sodium intake. By understanding the role of food in blood pressure control, individuals can take control of their health and reduce the risk of hypertension-related complications.

Impact of Diet on Blood Pressure

What we eat has a direct impact on our blood pressure. Certain foods can raise blood pressure by causing fluid retention or narrowing blood vessels, while others can help lower it by promoting better vascular health. For example, sodium, commonly found in processed foods and table salt, increases blood pressure by holding excess fluid in the body, adding stress to the heart and arteries. On the other hand, potassium helps to relax blood vessels and balance out the harmful effects of sodium.

Recent studies highlight that diets rich in fruits, vegetables, lean proteins, and whole grains, while low in saturated fats and processed sugars, can positively impact blood pressure. Scientific research emphasizes the importance of these dietary components, as they influence the body's electrolyte balance, blood volume, and blood vessel function, all key factors in hypertension management.

General Dietary Recommendations

A balanced diet is essential for controlling hypertension. Key recommendations include the following.

Fruits and Vegetables: These are high in fiber, vitamins, and minerals like potassium and magnesium, which help regulate blood pressure. One should aim for at least five servings of fruits and vegetables daily.

Whole Grains: Foods like brown rice, oats, and quinoa are rich in fiber and nutrients, offering better blood pressure control than refined grains such as white bread and pastries.

Lean Proteins: Incorporating lean meats like chicken, turkey, and fish, along with plant-based proteins such as beans, lentils, and tofu, helps maintain a healthy weight and reduces hypertension risk.

Low-Fat Dairy: Dairy products like yogurt and milk provide calcium, which has been linked to better blood pressure management.

Maintaining a healthy weight is another crucial aspect. Excess body weight, especially around the abdomen, can increase blood pressure. A balanced caloric intake, where the energy consumed matches the energy expended through activity, helps prevent obesity—a major risk factor for hypertension.

Specific Nutrients and Their Effects

Certain nutrients play a critical role in managing blood pressure.

Potassium: Potassium is a key nutrient in blood pressure management because it helps to counteract the effects of sodium. This mineral helps the body eliminate sodium and eases tension in blood vessel walls. Potassium balances amount of sodium in cells. Foods rich in potassium include apricots, bananas, cantaloupe, cherries, dates, figs, melon, kiwi, mango, nectarine, orange, papaya, prunes, fruit juices, potatoes, pumpkin, spinach, sweet potatoes, milk, tofu and yogurt.

Magnesium and Calcium: Known for its role in vascular health, magnesium helps regulate blood pressure by relaxing blood vessels. Foods like nuts, seeds, and leafy greens are great sources of magnesium. Calcium, on the other hand, supports the proper functioning of the heart and blood vessels. Foods like dairy products are rich in Calcium.

Omega-3 Fatty Acids: Found in fish such as salmon, mackerel, and sardines, omega-3 fatty acids reduce inflammation and improve cardiovascular function, contributing to lower blood pressure. Plant sources like flaxseeds and walnuts are also rich in them. These healthy fats can also help lower blood pressure by improving blood vessel function and reducing arterial stiffness.

DASH Diet

(Dietary Approaches to Stop Hypertension)

We have seen that diet is one of the most powerful tools in the fight against hypertension, and among the most effective dietary strategies is the **DASH** diet. The Dietary Approaches to Stop Hypertension diet is specifically designed to help lower blood pressure and improve heart health. Let us go through an overview of the DASH diet, its principles, effectiveness, and how to incorporate it into daily life.

Principles of the DASH Diet

The DASH diet is specifically designed to prevent and control high blood pressure. It is based on a simple yet powerful principle: eating a balanced diet rich in nutrients that support cardiovascular health while limiting those that can raise blood pressure. It emphasizes the following points.

<u>Fruits and Vegetables</u>: At least 4-5 servings of each per day to provide essential nutrients like potassium, fiber, and antioxidants while being low in calories and sodium.

<u>Whole Grains</u>: 6-8 servings per day, which supply fiber and nutrients that help regulate blood pressure. Foods like brown rice, whole wheat bread, and oatmeal are high in fiber and nutrients, which help maintain heart health and prevent blood pressure spikes.

<u>Lean Protein</u>: Incorporating 2 or fewer servings of lean meats, poultry, or fish per day. These are lower in saturated fat and cholesterol compared to red meat.

<u>Low-Fat Dairy</u>: 2-3 servings per day to provide calcium and vitamin D for better heart and vascular health.

<u>Nuts, Seeds, and Legumes</u>: 4-5 servings per week for added fiber, magnesium, and healthy fats.

<u>Sweets</u>: Restrict to 5 or fewer servings *per week*, opting for healthier alternatives

Multiple studies have shown that the DASH diet can significantly reduce blood pressure in just two weeks. It is particularly effective for individuals with stage 1 hypertension. In addition to lowering blood pressure, the

DASH diet improves overall heart health by lowering *LDL* (bad) cholesterol levels and reducing the risk of cardiovascular disease.

Compared to other diets, such as low-carb or ketogenic diets, the DASH diet offers a more sustainable approach to long-term health, as it focuses on nutrient-rich whole foods rather than excluding major food groups.

Making the DASH diet a part of daily life requires planning and creativity. Here are a few tips:

Meal Planning: Start by preparing weekly meal plans that incorporate a variety of fruits, vegetables, whole grains, and lean proteins. This ensures a balanced intake of essential nutrients.

Cooking Techniques: Opt for heart-healthy cooking methods such as grilling, steaming, or roasting instead of frying. Use olive oil or avocado oil instead of butter.

Sample Meal Plans

Given below are two sample meal plans for an ***American modification of the DASH diet***, including non-vegetarian and vegetarian options.

Non-Vegetarian DASH Meal Plan -American

Meal 1

Breakfast: Whole grain toast with avocado and a poached egg. A side of mixed berries and black coffee, tea or a glass of skim milk.

<u>Lunch</u>: Grilled turkey sandwich on whole wheat bread with spinach, tomato, and mustard. A side of baby carrots and hummus.

<u>Dinner</u>: Baked salmon with quinoa and roasted vegetables (zucchini, bell peppers, and asparagus).

<u>Snacks</u>: A small handful of unsalted almonds or low-fat yogurt.

Meal 2

<u>Breakfast</u>: Scrambled eggs with spinach and mushrooms, served with a whole wheat English muffin and a small orange.

<u>Lunch</u>: Grilled chicken salad with mixed greens, cherry tomatoes, cucumbers, and olive oil-lemon dressing. A small whole grain roll.

<u>Dinner</u>: Turkey meatballs in marinara sauce over whole wheat pasta, served with a side of steamed broccoli.

<u>Snacks</u>: Apple slices with peanut butter or a small handful of walnuts.

Vegetarian DASH Meal Plan - American

Meal 1

<u>Breakfast</u>: Steel-cut oatmeal with sliced bananas, flaxseeds, and a splash of almond milk.

<u>Lunch</u>: Quinoa salad with black beans, corn, avocado, and a lime vinaigrette dressing.

<u>Dinner</u>: Lentil soup with whole grain bread and a spinach salad with olive oil dressing.

Snacks: Low-fat Greek yogurt or air-popped popcorn.

Meal 2

Breakfast: Whole grain cereal with almond milk and fresh blueberries.

Lunch: Veggie wrap with hummus, cucumbers, shredded carrots, and spinach in a whole wheat tortilla.

Dinner: Stir-fried tofu with brown rice and mixed vegetables (broccoli, bell peppers, carrots) in a light soy sauce.

Snacks: Sliced cucumber and bell peppers with guacamole or hummus.

Below are given below two sample meal plans for **Indian modifications of the DASH diet,** including both non-vegetarian and vegetarian options to cater to the taste of Indians.

Non-Vegetarian DASH Meal Plan - Indian

Meal 1

Breakfast: Oats porridge with skimmed milk, topped with almonds and walnuts. One boiled egg and a small banana.

Lunch: Grilled chicken breast (spiced with turmeric and cumin), brown rice, sautéed spinach, and cucumber-tomato salad.

Dinner: Fish curry (made with minimal oil and spices), whole wheat chapati, and steamed broccoli with a squeeze of lemon.

Snacks: A handful of roasted chickpeas or unsalted peanuts.

Meal 2

Breakfast: Whole wheat toast with scrambled eggs and a glass of low-fat buttermilk.

Lunch: Baked salmon with lemon, quinoa, and stir-fried mixed vegetables (carrot, beans, capsicum).

Dinner: Chicken stew with sweet potatoes, brown rice, and a side of sautéed greens (spinach or kale).

Snacks: Low-fat yogurt with fresh fruits.

Vegetarian DASH Meal Plan - Indian

Meal 1

Breakfast: Ragi dosa with coconut chutney, one glass of unsweetened almond milk.

Lunch: Mixed vegetable curry (brinjal, cauliflower, peas) with brown rice and a green salad.

Dinner: Moong dal (green gram) curry, whole wheat chapati, and a side of boiled carrots and beans.

Snacks: Fresh fruit salad or a handful of unsalted almonds.

Meal 2

Breakfast: Vegetable upma (made with minimal oil) and a glass of low-fat milk.

Lunch: Rajma (kidney bean) curry, whole wheat chapati, and cucumber salad.

Dinner: Paneer bhurji (scrambled cottage cheese), brown rice, and a steamed broccoli and carrot salad.

Snacks: Roasted peanuts or a small portion of fresh fruits.

Numerous studies have demonstrated the effectiveness of the DASH diet in reducing blood pressure. When combined with lower sodium intake, the results were even more impressive, making the DASH diet one of the most effective dietary interventions for hypertension When compared to other dietary patterns, the DASH diet consistently ranks as one of the best for blood pressure management and overall heart health.

Salt Reduction Strategies

Sodium (**Na**) is a significant contributor to high blood pressure. Reducing sodium intake is one of the most effective ways to prevent and manage hypertension. Table salt is 40% sodium 60% chloride. The American Heart Association recommends limiting sodium intake to less than **2,300 mg** per day, which is roughly equivalent to one teaspoon of salt. An ideal target of **1,500 mg** is advised for individuals at risk of hypertension.

The typical US diet is high in salt (*Sodium chloride-* **NaCl**) and is mostly derived from processed food. Men consume about 10.7 gm of salt and women 7.3 g daily reports the Department of Agriculture and the Depot of Health and human services in USA. The daily recommend dose, however, is only 5.8 g salt (2300mg Na) for general population and 3.7 g (1500 mg Na) for those with hypertension.

It has been found in studies that over 50% of people are Salt Sensitive. The people who are sensitive to salt include:

- Those over the age of 65
- Overweight persons
- Those with diabetes
- Those with Chronic Kidney Disease (**CKD**)
- African Americans
- Women

<u>Simple strategies for reducing sodium include:</u>

Many processed and packaged foods contain hidden sodium. Always check nutrition labels for sodium content and aim for products labeled "low sodium" or "no added salt." Preparing meals at home allows better control over sodium intake. Use fresh ingredients and avoid adding excessive salt during cooking. Do not add salt to rice, pasta or hot cereals while cooking. Do not add salt on the table. Remove the salt shaker from the dining table. Remember, all salt – sea-salt and rock-salt are all still salt.

High salt foods that you should be wary of are Tomato Sauce, Soy sauce, other sauces, Pickles, Salad dressing, Bacon, Canned soups, Canned vegetables, Hot dogs, Cheese, salted butter and Ham. Also, select low salt canned food if inevitable. Use high salt condiments like ketchup, and mustard very sparingly. Snack on fresh fruits instead of salted crackers or chips. When eating out, ask less salt to be added.

In old age, taste decreases and hence the elderly will inadvertently add more salt. Similarly, the elderly, living alone may not be able to get fresh food. Hence they make good with canned and preserved food as they cannot cook by themselves.

Understanding the food labels by following the guidelines below is important.

- o Low sodium means < 140 mg of Na per serving.
- o Very low Sodium < 35 mg.
- o Sodium free is < 5 mg.
- o Reduced Sodium means 25% less than the original food item.
- o Light in Sodium means 50% less than original food item.
- o Unsalted / No salt added / Without added salt means no salt has been added to the food while processing.

<u>Healthy Substitutes</u>

Replacing high-sodium foods with healthier alternatives can make a big difference. When using canned vegetables, rinsing them under water can help remove some of the sodium. Instead of relying on salt for flavor, consider these healthy alternatives. Pickles like salted and spicy mangoes commonly used in India are high in salt content. It is ideal to avoid using them. If absolutely necessary, the mangoes may be washed in cold water and used avoiding the pickle juice.

Fresh herbs like basil, cilantro, and parsley, as well as spices such as paprika, cumin, and turmeric, can add depth and complexity to dishes instead of salt. Lemon juice or vinegar can enhance the taste of food and add a tangy kick, reducing the need for salt.

Hydration

Proper hydration is essential for overall health and blood pressure regulation. Drinking plenty of water helps maintain fluid balance, but it is important to limit caffeinated beverages and alcohol, as these can elevate blood pressure when consumed in excess.

Aim for at least 8-10 cups of water per day to stay hydrated. Alcohol intake should be moderated—no more than one drink per day for women and two drinks per day for men. Alcohol can raise blood pressure if consumed in large amounts.

Managing blood pressure is a long-term commitment. Regularly monitoring blood pressure at home can help individuals track their progress and adjust their diet as needed. It is also important to consult with healthcare providers and dietitians for personalized advice, especially when combining dietary changes with medication.

By following these dietary guidelines, incorporating the DASH diet, and reducing sodium intake, individuals can take significant steps toward managing and preventing hypertension. Proper nutrition, coupled with regular physical activity and lifestyle changes, forms the foundation of long-term heart health and blood pressure control.

Key Takeaways

- *Adopting a diet rich in fruits, vegetables, whole grains, lean proteins, and low-fat dairy while minimizing saturated fats, trans fats, and cholesterol can help manage and prevent high blood pressure.*

- *Key nutrients such as potassium, magnesium, calcium, and omega-3 fatty acids play crucial roles in regulating blood pressure. Incorporate foods high in these nutrients, like bananas, leafy greens, and fish, into your diet.*
- *The DASH diet is effective in reducing blood pressure and improving heart health. It emphasizes high intakes of fruits, vegetables, whole grains, lean proteins, and low-fat dairy while limiting saturated fats and red meat.*
- *Limiting sodium intake to less than 2,300 mg per day, with an ideal target of 1,500 mg for those with hypertension, is crucial for blood pressure management. Use herbs, spices, and acid-based flavorings as alternatives to salt.*
- *Adequate hydration supports overall health and aids in blood pressure management. Aim for 8-10 cups of water daily and moderate your intake of caffeinated and alcoholic beverages.*
- *Plan meals ahead to include DASH-friendly options, use healthy cooking methods, and read nutrition labels to avoid high-sodium foods.*
- *Regularly monitor blood pressure and consult healthcare providers or dietitians for personalized dietary advice and adjustments to maintain optimal blood pressure levels.*

Chapter 17 - PREVENTION OF HYPERTENSION

Hypertension is a major risk factor for heart disease, stroke, and kidney problems. Preventing hypertension is not only possible but essential for maintaining long-term health. This chapter focuses on simple, effective strategies to reduce the risk of developing hypertension, including a healthy diet, regular physical activity, weight management, and lifestyle changes like limiting alcohol and quitting smoking. By adopting these practices, individuals can lower their chances of hypertension and improve their overall well-being.

Hypertension significantly increases the risk of heart disease, stroke, and other serious health issues. Fortunately, hypertension is largely preventable through lifestyle choices and interventions.

Prevention strategies fall into three categories:

Primary Prevention, which focuses on avoiding the onset of high blood pressure.

Secondary Prevention, which aims to catch and manage early stages of hypertension.

Community And Public Health Initiatives that support widespread changes to reduce hypertension risks at a societal level.

Primary Prevention

Primary prevention is the cornerstone of avoiding hypertension. By making healthy lifestyle choices early on, individuals can significantly reduce their risk of developing high blood pressure. The focus is on long-term, sustainable habits that promote heart health.

Healthy Diet

One of the most important factors in preventing hypertension is maintaining a balanced, heart-healthy diet. The Dietary Approaches to Stop Hypertension (**DASH**) diet is a scientifically proven method of lowering blood pressure through nutrition. This eating plan emphasizes high intakes of fruits, vegetables, whole grains, and low-fat dairy products while limiting foods high in saturated fat and cholesterol. The DASH diet also encourages the consumption of lean proteins such as poultry, fish, and plant-based sources like beans and legumes. [See Chapter 16 on *Diet and Nutrition*].

Salt reduction plays a crucial role in managing blood pressure. The typical modern diet contains an excess of sodium, mainly due to processed and convenience foods. Reducing sodium intake to less than 2,300 mg per day, with an ideal limit of 1,500 mg for those at high risk of hypertension, can lead to substantial improvements in blood pressure. In addition to reducing sodium, increasing the intake of potassium and calcium is recommended. Foods such as bananas, oranges, spinach, and dairy products are rich in these nutrients, which help to balance the effects of sodium and relax blood vessels.

Physical Activity

Regular physical activity is a critical component of hypertension prevention. A distinction between physical activity and exercise must be understood. *Physical activity is any body movement that consumes calories like walking, climbing stairs, walking the dog, sweeping the floor and gardening. Exercise is a structured from of physical activity like jogging biking, swimming, weight lifting, yoga etc.*

The American Heart Association recommends that adults engage in at least 150 minutes of moderate-intensity aerobic exercise, such as brisk walking, or 75 minutes of vigorous-intensity exercise, such as running, each week. Exercise helps maintain a healthy weight, reduces arterial stiffness, and improves overall cardiovascular health, all of which are vital in preventing hypertension. Additionally, muscle-strengthening activities, such as weight lifting or yoga, should be incorporated at least twice a week.

Some of the important advantages of regular exercise are mentioned below.

o   Regular exercise can decrease BP by 5 – 7 mmHg.

- Exercise helps improve memory.
- It improves mood by releasing hormones named *Endorphins* which give a sense of well-being. They are called *"feel-good"* hormones because they can make the individual feel better and produce a positive state of mind.
- In diabetics, exercise helps reduce blood sugar.
- Exercise helps the individual to reduce weight and maintain ideal weight.
- Exercise reduces cancer risk.
- It increases the energy level in the body and increases stamina.
- It helps one sleep better.
- Exercise strengthens bones and makes them less liable to fractures.
- It improves cholesterol levels by reducing the bad (**LDL**) and raising the good (**HDL**) cholesterol levels.

Playing cricket, Practicing judo, karate, handball, racquetball, rowing, biking, playing rugby soccer or tennis, dancing and swimming are all aerobic exercises that are conducive to good health. Exercise helps us expend energy which is calculated in *Kilocalories* or *Calories. One Kilocalorie or Calorie is the amount of energy needed to raise the temp of a kilogram of water by 1 degree centigrade.* By exercising, the body burns fat and thus helps to reduce body weight. By expending 3500 Calories, one can burn a pound of fat.

Weight Management

Maintaining a healthy body weight is another essential factor in preventing hypertension. Obesity, particularly abdominal obesity, is strongly linked to an increased risk of developing high blood pressure.

Some of the exercises and the energy used up in Calories is given below.

Activity	Calories spent in 30 min	Calories spent in 60 min
Tennis	85	170
Walking - flat surface	120	240
Walking - uphill	162	324
Swimming	250	500
Basketball	282	564
Bicycling	283	566
Aerobic dance	342	684
Running	365	732

Achieving and sustaining a normal Body Mass Index (**BMI**) through a balanced diet and regular physical activity is crucial. Behavioral interventions such as self-monitoring, goal setting, and seeking social support are effective strategies in helping individuals manage their weight. These small, sustainable changes can make a big difference in long-term health outcomes.

Limiting Alcohol Intake

Excessive alcohol consumption is a known contributor to elevated blood pressure. To prevent hypertension, it is recommended that men limit their alcohol intake to no more than two drinks per day, and women to one drink per day. Alcohol, especially in large quantities, can raise blood pressure and interfere with the effectiveness of blood pressure medications. Moderation is the key to minimizing these risks.

Smoking Cessation

Smoking is harmful both to cardiovascular and lung health and is a contributing factor to hypertension. The chemicals in tobacco smoke damage the lining of blood vessels (*endothelium*), causing the arteries to narrow and increasing the risk of high blood pressure.

According to the CDC in 2021, approximately 28 million adults were smokers in the US. Worldwide it was estimated to be 2.2 billion in 2022. In the US 13% of white adults, 12% blacks, 8% Hispanic 5% Asians smoke. Every day about 2000 adolescents smoke their first cigarette and 300 will continue the habit thus adding to the population of smokes. Some of the harmful effects of smoking are:

- Higher risk of Lung cancer.
- Cancer in the mouth and throat and urinary bladder are commoner in smokers.
- The risk of Heart disease is very high.
- The risk of Stroke is high.
- Smokers run the risk of developing *Chronic Obstructive Pulmonary* (lung) *Disease* (**COPD**).
- In adolescents who smoke, the growth of the lungs is retarded.
- Smoking decreases the density of bones and thus contributes to fractures, especially in old women.
- Depression is often a consequence of smoking.
- Using Snuff and chewing tobacco, as is common in countries like India, is equally harmful.
- Second hand smoke or '*Passive smoking*' is dangerous especially for children in the family. The CDC has declared that approximately 41000 people die yearly due to second hand smoke of

which 7300 due to lung cancer and 34000 due to heart disease.

Quitting smoking can lead to immediate and long-term benefits, including lower blood pressure and improved heart health. Smoking cessation programs that include counseling, pharmacotherapy, and behavioral support can help individuals successfully quit and reduce their risk of developing hypertension. Quitting smoking needs a firm resolve. Smoking improves the overall fitness of the body and a feeling of increased energy. Some of the methods to stop smoking being advocated are:

- o Cutting back on caffeine as often smoking and drinking coffee go together.
- o Resolving to cut alcohol also as drinking alcohol is often accompanied by smoking.
- o Meditation, Yoga etc., are relaxation methods that help the smoker to quit.
- o Committing with one's friends regarding the resolve to stop smoking helps.
- o Avoiding people who smoke is equally important if one decides to quit the habit.
- o Finding other distractions like reading, exercising, watching a movie and gardening are quite helpful.
- o Drinking plenty of water is important if one decides to stop smoking.
- o Other methods to quit smoking are Nicotine gum, Nicotine lozenges, Nicotine patches, Nasal spray and inhalers. (Available only on prescription)
- o Some smoking-cessation medications like *Bupropion* and *Varenicline* available on

prescription only, help decrease withdrawal symptoms of smoking.

Secondary Prevention

Secondary prevention focuses on early detection and management of hypertension in individuals who are at risk or already have *Prehypertension* (elevated blood pressure that is not yet classified as hypertension). The goal is to prevent the condition from worsening and to avoid complications.

Early Detection

Early detection of elevated blood pressure is essential for preventing the progression to full-blown hypertension. Screening recommendations suggest that individuals with risk factors, such as a family history of hypertension, obesity, diabetes, or other cardiovascular conditions, should have their blood pressure checked regularly. Healthcare providers will also look for other indicators, such as high cholesterol or signs of metabolic syndrome.

Early identification of high blood pressure allows for interventions at a stage when lifestyle changes can still be effective. The criteria for diagnosing Prehypertension and Stage 1 Hypertension are well-established, focusing on blood pressure readings and assessing cardiovascular risk factors. Accurate measurement and repeated assessments are important in making a correct diagnosis.

Lifestyle Modifications

Once elevated blood pressure is detected, lifestyle modifications similar to those used in primary prevention are often the first line of defense. Dietary changes, such as reducing sodium intake, increasing potassium consumption, and following the DASH diet, are recommended. Regular physical activity and weight management also play key roles in controlling blood pressure at this stage. These interventions are typically sufficient for individuals with prehypertension or mild hypertension, though more intensive treatment may be required if blood pressure continues to rise.

Adherence to Medication

For individuals diagnosed with hypertension, medication adherence is critical to preventing the condition from worsening and reducing the risk of complications such as heart disease and stroke. Non-adherence to medication regimens is a common issue that can lead to uncontrolled hypertension and increase the risk of severe health problems. Taking blood pressure medications as prescribed, even if one feels well, is crucial to maintaining a stable blood pressure.

Physicians may prescribe antihypertensive medications, such as ACE inhibitors, angiotensin II receptor blockers (ARBs), or diuretics, to help lower blood pressure. Initially, a single drug may be started in a small dose and the dose stepped up till the blood pressure reaches the target goals for the patient. Patients must be educated about the importance of sticking to their treatment plan and regularly monitoring their blood pressure at home. Support from healthcare professionals, family members, and online resources can help patients stay on track with their medications.

Community and Public Health Initiatives

While individual choices are key to preventing hypertension, community and public health initiatives can play a significant role in supporting these efforts. These initiatives aim to create environments that encourage healthier lifestyles and make it easier for people to adopt and sustain the behaviors that prevent hypertension.

- Public Education Campaigns: Public education campaigns can raise awareness about hypertension, promote healthy behaviors, and encourage regular screenings. Health literacy initiatives provide individuals with knowledge to make informed health decisions.
- Mass Media Campaigns: Television and radio campaigns can inform the public about hypertension risks, preventive measures, and the importance of blood pressure checks. Social media platforms like Facebook, Instagram, and Twitter can be used to share facts, tips, and engage users through hashtags like #FightHypertension.
- Health Education in Schools: Students can be taught about healthy eating and physical activity, with schools collaborating with healthcare providers for screenings. Implementing healthier school meal programs helps establish lifelong habits that prevent hypertension.

Arjun, a 24-year-old software engineer, led a sedentary lifestyle, spending long hours at his desk. During a routine medical checkup organized by his company, he was surprised to learn that his blood pressure was slightly elevated at 130/85 mmHg, a condition known as prehypertension. This came as a concern to Arjun, given that both his parents were hypertensive. Although his blood pressure was not yet in the dangerous range, his physician explained that without intervention, Arjun could develop full-blown hypertension in the future.

The doctor emphasized the importance of early lifestyle modifications to prevent further elevation in his blood pressure. Arjun was advised to adopt a healthier diet, focusing on reducing salt intake and eating more fruits and vegetables. Regular physical activity, such as brisk walking or light gym workouts for at least 30 minutes a day, was strongly encouraged. Managing stress, whether through meditation or yoga, and maintaining a healthy weight were also highlighted as key measures. The physician also suggested that Arjun avoid excessive caffeine and alcohol, both of which could contribute to higher blood pressure.

Motivated by this wake-up call, Arjun made gradual changes to his lifestyle, determined to keep his blood pressure under control and prevent future complications.

- <u>Community Workshops and Health Fairs</u>: Free blood pressure screenings in accessible locations can be paired with educational workshops. Community leaders and local figures should be involved to encourage participation and spread awareness.

- <u>Mobile Health Applications and Digital Tools</u>: Apps that monitor blood pressure and text messaging programs that send health tips can be promoted. Virtual classes and webinars on hypertension management provide ongoing support.
- <u>Workplace Wellness Programs</u>: Employers can offer free blood pressure screenings, educational resources, and stress management initiatives. Physical activity challenges and healthy snack options should be encouraged.
- <u>Collaborate with Healthcare Providers</u>: Healthcare professionals can provide patient education on lifestyle changes and medication adherence. Educational materials in clinics and group sessions can help patients with self-monitoring techniques.
- <u>Health Initiatives in Religious Institutions</u>: Blood pressure screenings and health workshops in religious spaces can effectively reach communities. Religious leaders can promote health as part of spiritual well-being.
- <u>Public Health Announcements and Text Alerts</u>: Public transportation systems like trains and buses and emergency alert systems can be used to notify the public about hypertension screenings and educational campaigns.
- <u>Culturally Tailored Messaging</u>: Educational materials should be created in multiple languages, incorporating traditional diets and practices. Culturally relevant celebrities and community leaders can be used to endorse healthy habits.

- <u>Hypertension Awareness Events</u>: Designated awareness days or weeks can be organized with screenings and media coverage. Public figures and social media campaigns can help spread awareness and encourage healthy competition around hypertension prevention.

These methods aim to provide accessible information and practical resources to help individuals prevent hypertension, fostering greater awareness and encouraging healthy lifestyle changes across populations.

These public education methods, when implemented effectively, can have a profound impact on reducing the burden of hypertension by fostering greater awareness and encouraging healthy lifestyle changes across populations. The goal is to provide accessible, understandable information to people of all ages and backgrounds, empowering them to take control of their cardiovascular health. Community-based programs can provide individuals with practical resources and support to prevent hypertension. Given below are a few examples of community-based programs that can provide practical resources and support to prevent hypertension.

National Diabetes Prevention Program (NDPP)

Although initially focused on diabetes prevention, the NDPP helps prevent hypertension by promoting healthy lifestyle changes.

Million Hearts® Initiative

A national initiative by the CDC and Centers for Medicare & Medicaid Services (CMS) to prevent 1 million heart attacks and strokes within five years.

Faith-based Health Promotion Programs

Churches, mosques, and other faith communities offer health education programs that focus on managing and preventing hypertension.

Worksite Wellness Programs

Many employers implement wellness programs to promote heart health and prevent hypertension among employees.

Hypertension Control Program (HCP) by Community Health Centers

Community health centers in underserved areas often run Hypertension Control Programs to target at-risk populations.

These community-based programs are critical in providing the tools and education necessary for preventing and managing hypertension, often leveraging local resources to create accessible and sustainable health interventions.

Partnerships between healthcare providers, local organizations, schools, and businesses can thus help create supportive environments that encourage healthy choices. Community gardens, walking groups, and wellness challenges are examples of local interventions that promote healthier lifestyles and prevent hypertension.

Policy Initiatives

Government and healthcare policymakers can reduce hypertension rates through various strategies aimed at promoting healthier environments. Here are several effective methods:

- <u>Access to Healthy Foods</u>: Access to fruits and vegetables can be improved by subsidizing them, making healthy food more affordable. Healthier school lunch programs, food labeling laws, and sugary drink taxes should be promoted. Support for urban agriculture and community gardens in underserved areas will enhance access to fresh produce.

- <u>Sodium Reduction</u>: Sodium reduction in processed foods can be achieved by setting targets for the food industry and mandating sodium labeling. Advertising high-sodium foods to children should be regulated. Lowering sodium intake has been proven to reduce population-wide blood pressure levels.

- <u>Promotion of Physical Activity</u>: More parks, walking paths, and bike lanes should be created to encourage physical activity. Schools should implement daily physical education programs. Regular physical activity is essential for lowering blood pressure and managing weight, both crucial in preventing hypertension.

- <u>Public Health Education</u>: Public awareness campaigns on hypertension risks and blood pressure monitoring should be enhanced. Hypertension screening in pharmacies, workplaces, and community centers must be promoted to increase awareness and early intervention.

- <u>Healthcare Access</u>: Access to primary care services should be expanded in underserved areas. Coverage for hypertension screening and management should be mandated, and team-based care models can help manage hypertension. Early detection and consistent management are key to lowering hypertension rates.

- <u>Regulation of Smoking and Alcohol</u>: Increased taxes on tobacco and alcohol, along with smoking bans in public spaces, should be implemented. Limiting advertising of alcohol and tobacco, especially to young people, will reduce hypertension risks.

- <u>Healthier Workplaces</u>: Workplace wellness programs focused on hypertension screening, health education, and stress management should be encouraged. Healthier food options in workplace cafeterias and flexible work hours can foster a less stressful environment.

- <u>Tobacco Control</u>: Anti-tobacco regulations should be strengthened, and smoking cessation programs made more accessible. Reducing tobacco use is critical in lowering hypertension and cardiovascular disease risks.

- <u>Safe Housing</u>: Improving housing conditions, particularly by addressing noise pollution and overcrowding, will help reduce stress and hypertension. Housing policies should ensure low-income families have access to healthcare, healthy food, and safe spaces for physical activity.

- <u>Environmental Regulation</u>: Stricter air quality regulations and clean energy initiatives should be enforced to reduce exposure to pollutants, improving cardiovascular health and reducing hypertension risk.

These policies, implemented at the national and local levels, can create healthier environments and promote long-term prevention of hypertension by addressing lifestyle and environmental factors.

The Government of India initiated a National Program for Prevention and Control of Cancer, Diabetes, Cardiovascular Diseases and Stroke (**NPCDCS**) in 2010-11. It is a national government program to improve screening and treatment for NCDs. The India Hypertension Control Initiative (**IHCI**) is a government-led program that aims to reduce the prevalence of hypertension in India.

Additionally, ensuring that individuals have access to care is essential for effective hypertension prevention. This means improving access to regular blood pressure screening, medications, and lifestyle counseling, particularly in underserved communities where healthcare resources may be limited.

Research and Evaluation

Ongoing research is crucial for developing and refining strategies to prevent hypertension. Researchers continue to study the most effective interventions, including new medications, public health initiatives, and community-based programs.

Regular evaluation of programs and policies ensures they are meeting their goals and making a real impact. This includes assessing the effectiveness of sodium reduction efforts, physical activity promotion, and screening initiatives. With a data-driven approach, public health officials can make necessary adjustments to ensure the best possible outcomes for the community.

In conclusion, preventing hypertension requires a multifaceted approach that includes individual efforts, healthcare support, and community-based interventions. By adopting a healthy lifestyle and supporting public health initiatives, we can work together to reduce the burden of hypertension and improve cardiovascular health for everyone.

Key Takeaways

- *Adopting the DASH diet, reducing sodium intake, and increasing potassium and calcium-rich foods are essential for maintaining healthy blood pressure levels.*
- *Regular physical activity, including at least 150 minutes of moderate-intensity exercise per week, helps reduce the risk of hypertension and improves overall cardiovascular health.*
- *Maintaining a healthy weight through balanced nutrition and physical activity is key to preventing and managing hypertension.*
- *Moderating alcohol consumption, with a maximum of one drink per day for women and two for men, helps reduce the risk of developing high blood pressure.*
- *Quitting smoking is vital for improving cardiovascular health and lowering the risk of hypertension.*
- *Regular blood pressure screening, especially for those with risk factors, is crucial for early intervention and preventing the progression of hypertension.*

- *Long-term changes in diet, exercise, and stress management can help manage prehypertension and prevent it from advancing to full-blown hypertension.*
- *Following prescribed medication regimens is essential for controlling hypertension and preventing complications.*
- *Community programs, public health policies, and education campaigns play a vital role in spreading awareness, improving access to care, and promoting healthy behaviors to prevent hypertension.*

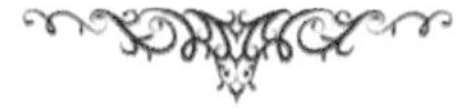

Chapter 18 - LIVING WITH HYPERTENSION

Living with hypertension does not mean one has to sacrifice a full, active life. By making simple adjustments to one's daily routine—such as taking medications as prescribed, adopting a healthy diet, exercising regularly, and managing stress— an individual can effectively control his blood pressure. This chapter provides practical strategies for managing hypertension, maintaining mental well-being, and finding support, all while highlighting real-life stories of individuals who have successfully managed their condition and improved their quality of life.

Hypertension, or high blood pressure, is a chronic condition that requires consistent management. With proper medication adherence, lifestyle adjustments, and emotional support, many individuals successfully manage their condition. Let us discuss the practical strategies for day-to-day management, ways to cope with the mental and emotional challenges of hypertension, and real-life testimonials from people who are thriving despite their diagnosis. Let us explore how to live well with high blood pressure.

Day-to-Day Management:

Managing hypertension is not about occasional efforts; it is about incorporating healthy practices into your daily routine. By being mindful of your medication, diet, exercise, and lifestyle choices, you can control your blood pressure and prevent complications. Let us break down the key areas of daily management.

Adherence to Medication

One of the cornerstones of managing hypertension is consistent medication use. Missing doses or stopping medication without medical advice can lead to dangerously high blood pressure and increase the risk of heart disease, stroke, or kidney damage. Studies have shown that people who adhere to their medication regimen have better blood pressure management and a lower risk of complications. According to Muntner (2022), adhering to prescribed antihypertensive medications reduces these risks and helps maintain blood pressure within a healthy range.

Improving medication adherence can be as simple as using a pill organizer that separates doses by day and time or setting daily reminders on your phone. Understanding why each medication is prescribed can also increase adherence. Ask your healthcare provider about how the medications work and what to expect from them. When patients understand the purpose and benefits of their medication, they are more likely to take it consistently.

Monitoring Blood Pressure

Regular home blood pressure monitoring is an essential part of managing hypertension. It allows you to track your progress and alert your healthcare provider to any significant changes. Monitoring your blood pressure at home also gives a more accurate picture of your health, as it avoids "white coat syndrome" — when blood pressure spikes while visiting the doctor.

Choosing the right blood pressure monitor is crucial. Look for devices that are easy to use, accurate, and approved by healthcare authorities. Your doctor will be able to advise you on the choice of an appropriate BP monitor. The American Heart Association recommends upper-arm monitors over wrist or finger devices for more reliable readings. Ensure you measure your blood pressure roughly at the same time each day, and always follow the manufacturer's instructions for use. Make sure you know how to use the monitor correctly—this includes sitting quietly for a few minutes before taking a reading and keeping your arm at heart level. [See Chapter 5 on *Blood Pressure Measurement*].

Diet and Exercise

Diet has already been dealt with in detail in Chapter 16. A healthy diet is one of the most effective ways to manage your blood pressure. The DASH diet is specifically designed to lower blood pressure. Appel and colleagues have reported that following the DASH diet significantly reduced blood pressure within just a few weeks.

Regular physical activity helps strengthen your heart and lower blood pressure. Aerobic exercises like walking, swimming, or cycling are particularly effective. Cornelissen & Smart in 2013 demonstrated that even moderate exercise, when performed consistently, can lead to long-term blood pressure control. Aiming for at least 150 minutes of moderate-intensity exercise per week, is recommended by health experts.

Lifestyle Adjustments

<u>Weight Management</u>:   Maintaining a healthy weight is crucial for lowering blood pressure. Excess weight, particularly around the abdomen, puts extra strain on your heart and can lead to higher blood pressure. Sacks and colleagues in a 2009 study found that losing even a small amount of weight can make a significant difference in blood pressure control. If you are overweight, losing as little as 5 to 10 pounds can help reduce your blood pressure and lower your risk of other health problems.

<u>Alcohol and Smoking</u>:   Both excessive alcohol consumption and smoking can worsen hypertension. Limiting alcohol to moderate levels (no more than one drink per day for women and two for men) can reduce blood pressure. Meanwhile, quitting smoking has immediate and long-term benefits for heart health. Muller and colleagues emphasize that even cutting down on alcohol and tobacco can yield positive effects on blood pressure management.

Coping Strategies: Managing Stress and Mental Health

Living with hypertension can be stressful, and stress itself can raise blood pressure temporarily. Therefore, finding effective ways to manage stress and maintain mental well-being is essential for overall health.

> *Maria, a 28-year-old accountant at a large multinational bank, was under immense stress due to the heavy workload she faced. Her responsibilities extended beyond normal working hours, often spilling over into weekends and holidays. Despite her best efforts, she found it nearly impossible to visit her aging parents or take time off. To meet the constant deadlines imposed by her manager, Maria frequently worked late into the night and was often woken early in the morning to complete urgent tasks. This relentless pressure left her sleep-deprived and skipping meals regularly.*
>
> *After months of enduring this, Maria began experiencing frequent headaches, fatigue, and anxiety. Concerned, she consulted her family physician, who discovered her blood pressure was dangerously high at 176/114 mmHg. She was immediately put on antihypertensive medication and advised to address her overwork situation. Fortunately, when she spoke to her senior manager, he responded with understanding and adjusted her workload.*
>
> *Maria began following her doctor's recommendations, adhering to her medication, and making time for recreation and rest. As a result, her blood pressure gradually came under control, and her stress levels significantly decreased, allowing her to maintain a healthier work-life balance.*

Here are some strategies to help you cope. When you feel stressed, try taking a few slow, deep breaths—inhale deeply through your nose, hold for a moment, and then exhale slowly through your mouth.

Stress Management Techniques

Incorporating relaxation methods into your daily routine can help lower stress and, in turn, reduce blood pressure. Deep breathing exercises, progressive muscle relaxation, and meditation are simple techniques that can be practiced anywhere. Relaxation techniques reduce the body's stress response, leading to lower blood pressure levels over time.

<u>Mindfulness and Yoga</u>: Yoga and mindfulness practices have shown promising results in reducing both stress and blood pressure. These methods promote relaxation while improving focus and self-awareness. Cramer and colleagues in 2014 reported that yoga specifically has a positive impact on heart rate variability, which is a marker of cardiovascular health. Yoga in addition has exercises (*Asanas*) which help increase muscle tone, flexibility and balance.

Mindfulness involves focusing on the present moment without judgment, helping you to manage your thoughts and emotions more effectively. Even just a few minutes of mindfulness meditation each day can make a difference. Including even short sessions of yoga or mindfulness meditation in your daily routine can help manage hypertension.

Mental Health Support

<u>Counseling and Therapy</u>:   Living with a chronic condition like hypertension can lead to anxiety, depression, or feelings of frustration. Accessing mental health support through counseling or therapy can provide valuable tools for coping with these emotions. Psychological interventions, such as cognitive-behavioral therapy (**CBT**), can help reduce both anxiety and blood pressure. Do not hesitate to seek professional help if you need it—taking care of your mental health is just as important as managing your physical health.

<u>Support Groups</u>:   Sharing your experience with others who understand your challenges can provide emotional support and encouragement. Support groups, whether in-person or online, offer a safe space to discuss concerns, exchange tips, and gain reassurance. Patients who participate in support groups experience improved mental well-being and better health outcomes.

Balancing Life with Hypertension

<u>Work and Social Life</u>:   Managing a chronic condition like hypertension while maintaining a busy work and social life can be challenging. Living with hypertension does not mean you have to give up the activities you enjoy or let your condition dominate your life. However, with the right strategies, it is possible to balance both. Communication is key — talk to your employer about any health accommodations you may need, such as flexible work hours or a stress-free work environment. An open dialogue with employers and colleagues can help reduce workplace stress and make it easier to manage your health.

<u>Self-Care Practices</u>: Self-care is crucial for long-term health management. Prioritize adequate sleep, relaxation, and hobbies that bring you joy. Aim for 7-9 hours of restful sleep each night, as poor sleep can raise your blood pressure. Regular relaxation is also crucial; whether it is taking a warm bath, reading a book, or enjoying a hobby, make time for activities that help you unwind.

The importance of self-care in reducing stress and improving overall quality of life cannot be overemphasized. Making time for yourself, even for small activities, can help you manage hypertension more effectively. Self-care is not just about physical relaxation; it is also about nurturing your emotional and mental health, so engage in activities that bring you joy and fulfillment.

Personal Stories:

Real-life experiences from people living with hypertension can provide valuable insights and inspiration. These stories highlight that with the right approach, living well with high blood pressure is entirely possible. Remember, *managing hypertension is a marathon, not a sprint—small, consistent changes can lead to big results*.

Many individuals have successfully managed their hypertension through a combination of medication, lifestyle changes, and emotional support. These success stories highlight that hypertension can be controlled with dedication and consistency.

People who have taken control of their hypertension often describe how it positively changed their lives. Living with hypertension is not without its challenges. Many individuals face setbacks, whether it is difficulty adhering to medication, maintaining a healthy lifestyle, or dealing with the emotional toll of a chronic condition. Learning from these struggles can provide valuable insights for others in similar situations.

The path to successful hypertension management often involves trial and error. These stories offer practical tips and encouragement for anyone navigating the complexities of living with hypertension.

Encouraging Community Involvement

<u>Support Networks</u>:   Family, friends, and the broader community play a crucial role in supporting those with hypertension. The importance of a strong support network for managing chronic health conditions is to be emphasized. Simple acts of encouragement or assistance from loved ones can make a significant difference in maintaining healthy habits.

<u>Engagement in Local Initiatives</u>: Getting involved in local health initiatives or support groups can provide additional encouragement and resources for managing hypertension. Individuals should be encouraged to participate in local events, such as community health screenings or fitness groups, which can offer both social interaction and health benefits.

Living with hypertension thus requires a proactive approach, but it is entirely possible to lead a full and active life with the right strategies in place. By adhering to medication, making lifestyle changes, managing stress, and seeking support when needed, you can control your blood pressure and live well. Take inspiration from those who have faced the same challenges and succeeded

— their stories remind us that hypertension does not have to limit your life.

Key Takeaways

- *Medication adherence is essential for controlling blood pressure and preventing complications; use strategies like pill organizers and reminders to stay on track.*
- *Regular blood pressure monitoring at home helps track progress and detect any changes, ensuring timely adjustments to your treatment plan.*
- *A healthy diet, such as the DASH diet, and regular physical exercise are effective ways to manage hypertension and may reduce the need for medication.*
- *Stress management techniques, including meditation, deep breathing, and yoga, can lower stress and help keep blood pressure in check.*
- *Mental health support, such as therapy and support groups, can provide emotional relief and improve overall well-being for individuals living with hypertension.*
- *Lifestyle adjustments like weight management, limiting alcohol, and quitting smoking significantly contribute to better blood pressure control.*
- *A strong support network of family, friends, and community resources is key to managing hypertension and maintaining long-term health.*

Chapter 19 - MYTHS AND MISCONCEPTIONS ABOUT HYPERTENSION

Hypertension, or high blood pressure, is a common condition surrounded by many myths and misconceptions. These misunderstandings can prevent people from effectively managing their blood pressure or seeking the right treatment. In this chapter, we will attempt to debunk some of the most prevalent myths about hypertension and clarify the facts with scientific evidence. By dispelling these misconceptions, you will gain a clearer understanding of how to take control of your health and manage hypertension more effectively.

When it comes to hypertension, there is no shortage of myths and misconceptions. These misunderstandings can prevent individuals from taking the necessary steps to manage their blood pressure effectively. We will demystify some common myths surrounding hypertension and clarify these misunderstandings with scientific evidence. By the end, you will have a clearer understanding of hypertension and be equipped to make more informed decisions about your health.

4 Common Myths Debunked

Hypertension is one of the most common health conditions globally, yet misinformation about it continues to circulate. Misconceptions can lead to ineffective management or even neglect of treatment. Let us take a look at some of the most prevalent myths and set the record straight.

Myth 1: Hypertension Only Affects Older Adults

Many people believe that hypertension is a disease of the elderly. While it is true that the likelihood of developing high blood pressure increases with age, it is a baseless misconception that young people are immune to the condition.

Clarification: Hypertension can affect people of all ages, including teenagers and young adults. Factors such as obesity, high sodium intake, physical inactivity, and even genetic predisposition can lead to high blood pressure in younger individuals. With the rising prevalence of unhealthy lifestyles, younger people are increasingly being diagnosed with hypertension. Early onset hypertension is becoming more common, especially in individuals with poor diet, lack of exercise, and higher body weight.

Myth 2: Hypertension is Just a Result of Stress

Stress or "tension" is often blamed for hypertension, but while it can cause a temporary spike in blood pressure, it is not the sole or primary cause of chronic hypertension. The relationship between stress and high blood pressure is more nuanced than many realize. Many successful people have HTN which they keep under control with their lifestyle modifications and appropriate medication.

Clarification: Chronic hypertension is typically caused by a combination of genetic, lifestyle, and physiological factors, not just stress. While stress can temporarily raise blood pressure, it is long-term factors such as poor diet, lack of physical activity, and genetic predisposition that lead to sustained high blood pressure. While managing stress is important, relying on stress reduction alone without addressing diet, exercise, and other risk factors is insufficient for managing hypertension.

Myth 3: Only People with HBP Need to Monitor Their BP

Many people assume that unless they have been diagnosed with hypertension, they do not need to check their blood pressure regularly. This is a dangerous misconception.

Clarification: Monitoring your blood pressure is important for everyone, especially if you have risk factors such as a family history of hypertension, obesity, or a sedentary lifestyle. High blood pressure can be asymptomatic for years, making it critical to monitor blood pressure levels regularly to catch any early signs of elevated readings. The importance of regular monitoring to prevent the onset of hypertension and identify issues before they become severe has been emphasized in many studies.

Myth 4: All Hypertension Medications Cause Significant Side Effects

Concerns about the side effects of blood pressure medications can deter people from taking the medication they need. This misconception can result in patients neglecting their treatment plan, potentially leading to severe health complications.

<u>Clarification</u>   While some older medications were known for significant side effects, newer antihypertensive medications are generally well-tolerated. The side effects of modern medications are often mild and manageable. Additionally, healthcare providers can customize treatment plans to minimize side effects, making medication a safe and effective part of managing hypertension. Advances in pharmacology have led to the development of drugs that provide effective blood pressure control with fewer unwanted side effects.

Fact vs. Fiction

To effectively manage hypertension, it is important to separate fact from fiction. Here, we address some common misunderstandings with solid scientific evidence. This will help you better understand the condition and make informed decisions about your health.

> *David, a 30-year-old businessman, was diagnosed with hypertension and initially managed well on appropriate medications prescribed by his physician. His blood pressure remained under control for some time. However, during a chance meeting with an old school friend, David was wrongly advised that long-term use of antihypertensive medication could damage his kidneys, and that simple salt restriction was sufficient to control blood pressure. Trusting this advice, David stopped taking his medications and did not consult his doctor for the next seven years, as he had no apparent symptoms.*
>
> *One morning, David was found unconscious in his bathroom and was rushed to the hospital. Upon arrival, doctors diagnosed that he had suffered a stroke. His blood pressure was dangerously high at 210/136 mmHg. David was immediately admitted to the ICU and received intensive care. After a week in the hospital, he was discharged but with residual weakness and disability on the left side of his body, requiring extensive physical therapy for recovery.*
>
> *The doctors restarted David on antihypertensive medications and strongly warned him to adhere to the prescribed treatment to prevent another life-threatening event.*

Fact 1: Hypertension is Often Asymptomatic

One of the most dangerous aspects of hypertension is that it often presents no symptoms. People may feel perfectly healthy even as their blood pressure rises to dangerous levels.

<u>Clarification</u>:   Hypertension is often called the *"Silent Killer"* because most individuals with high blood pressure do not experience any symptoms. This lack of symptoms can make it easy to ignore or remain unaware of the condition until it reaches a critical stage, increasing the risk of heart attack, stroke, and other serious complications. Regular check-ups and blood pressure monitoring are crucial for early detection. Lack of symptoms underscores the importance of routine health screenings for early intervention.

Fact 2: Lifestyle Changes Can Significantly Lower Blood Pressure

A common misconception is that medication is the only way to control hypertension. However, lifestyle modifications can make a significant impact on blood pressure levels.

<u>Clarification</u>:   Dietary changes, regular exercise, weight management, and reducing alcohol intake are proven ways to lower blood pressure. The diet, for instance, has been shown to reduce blood pressure significantly. In some cases, lifestyle changes alone can bring blood pressure back to normal levels, eliminating the need for medication. Such lifestyle changes can be as effective as medication for many patients, making them a key part of hypertension management. When lifestyle changes are supplemented with medication, the dose of medication can be considerably reduced to control the high blood pressure.

Fact 3: Blood Pressure Can Fluctuate Throughout the Day

It is a common belief that once you have a single high blood pressure reading, it is indicative of hypertension. But blood pressure naturally fluctuates throughout the day due to various factors.

<u>Clarification</u>: Blood pressure rises and falls depending on activities, emotions, and time of day. For example, it tends to be lower when you are at rest and higher when you are active or stressed. Understanding these natural fluctuations is important for accurate diagnosis and management. This daily pattern, known as *'Diurnal Variation'*, is completely normal. However, if your blood pressure does not dip at night or if it spikes too much during certain activities, it could indicate a problem. Blood pressure should always be measured under consistent conditions to obtain reliable readings, and multiple measurements over time give a better overall picture of one's blood pressure health.

Fact 4: Not All Hypertension is Caused by Lifestyle Factors

Another common belief is that hypertension is always the result of unhealthy lifestyle choices, but this is not entirely accurate.

<u>Clarification</u>: It is important to recognize that hypertension is a complex condition with multiple causes. While poor lifestyle choices like a high-sodium diet, smoking, and lack of physical activity contribute to hypertension, genetics and underlying medical conditions also play a significant role. Secondary hypertension, for example, is caused by conditions like

kidney disease or hormonal disorders and requires different treatment approaches. Both genetic predisposition and environmental factors work together to influence blood pressure, making it important to consider both when managing hypertension.

Patient Education & Informed Decisions

Beyond debunking myths and presenting the facts, empowering individuals with the knowledge they need to make informed decisions about their health is essential. Here is how patients can take control of their hypertension management.

Understanding Blood Pressure Readings

Blood pressure readings consist of two numbers: systolic and diastolic pressure. The first number (*Systolic*) measures the pressure in your arteries when your heart contracts, while the second number (*Diastolic*) measures the pressure in your arteries when your heart relaxes and is at rest between beats. It is crucial to understand what these numbers mean, and which ranges are considered healthy or hypertensive. Being able to interpret these numbers helps you track your health and take timely action. [See Chapter 5 on *Blood Pressure Measurement*].

Empowering Patients to Ask Questions

Managing hypertension is not just about taking medication or following a diet; it is also about being actively involved in your healthcare. One of the most important things you can do is ask questions when you visit your healthcare provider. Many patients feel intimidated when discussing their condition with healthcare providers. However, asking the right questions can lead to better understanding and more personalized care.

Do not hesitate to ask your doctor questions about your diagnosis, medication, and treatment plan. Some helpful questions include:

- "What are my blood pressure numbers, and what do they mean for my health?"

- "How can lifestyle changes help me manage hypertension?"

- "Are there side effects I should watch out for with my medication?"

- "How often should I monitor my blood pressure at home?"

- "If I find a high reading when monitoring at home, what should I do?"

Good communication with your healthcare provider can lead to better outcomes and help you feel more confident in managing your hypertension.

Using Reliable Resources

In today's digital age, it is important to access credible sources of information about hypertension. Not all information found online is accurate or trustworthy. Also, one should be wary of friends and acquaintances giving unsolicited advice regarding the treatment. Reliable resources include websites like the *American*

Heart Association and books written by medical professionals with expertise in cardiovascular health.

<u>Resource List</u>: A few reputable sources include:

American   Heart   Association: www.heart.org

Centers for Disease Control and Prevention (CDC): www.cdc.gov

Mayo   Clinic: www.mayoclinic.org

Promoting Regular Monitoring and Follow-Up

Regular monitoring is essential for managing hypertension. Home blood pressure monitors are a valuable tool for tracking your readings between doctor visits.

Follow up with your physician regularly, especially if you have been diagnosed with hypertension. This ensures that your treatment plan is working and that your condition remains under control. Monitoring and maintaining a blood pressure journal allows your doctor to adjust your treatment plan as necessary.

By understanding the facts and myths about hypertension, patients can make informed decisions about their health. Knowledge is the key to taking control of high blood pressure and preventing its serious complications.

Key Takeaways

- *Hypertension can affect all ages, not just older adults—factors like obesity and sedentary lifestyles increase the risk in younger people.*
- *Stress alone does not cause chronic hypertension; it is usually a combination of genetic, lifestyle, and physiological factors.*
- *Regular blood pressure monitoring is important for everyone, not just those already diagnosed with hypertension, to detect early signs.*
- *Modern hypertension medications are generally well-tolerated with minimal side effects, and treatment plans can be customized to suit individual needs.*
- *Hypertension is often asymptomatic, making regular check-ups crucial for early detection and management.*
- *Lifestyle changes, such as adopting a healthier diet and exercising, can significantly lower blood pressure and reduce the need for medication.*
- *Blood pressure fluctuates naturally throughout the day, so regular monitoring under consistent conditions is essential for accurate management.*
- *Not all hypertension is caused by lifestyle choices; genetics and underlying medical conditions can also contribute to high blood pressure.*

Chapter 20 - RESOURCES AND SUPPORT GROUPS

Managing hypertension can feel overwhelming, but one does not have to face it alone. Support groups and reliable resources provide crucial help on the journey to better health. This chapter explores how connecting with others, whether through local meetups or online communities, can offer emotional and practical support. Additionally, you will discover trusted books, websites, and organizations that provide up-to-date information, empowering you to stay informed and advocate for your own health. By accessing the right resources and joining a supportive community, managing hypertension becomes a shared and more manageable experience.

Managing high blood pressure can often feel like a solitary journey. But it does not have to be so. Whether you are a patient or a caregiver, finding support and reliable information is crucial in managing hypertension effectively. Here we discuss practical guidance on tapping into resources, joining support groups, and empowering yourself with the right tools to stay informed and proactive. Let us dive into the importance of support, where to find it, and how to advocate for yourself as a hypertension patient.

Finding Support

Importance of Community and Online Support Groups

Living with hypertension can be overwhelming at times. Support groups can play a vital role in helping individuals cope, not only through emotional comfort but also by providing practical advice. Research indicates that support groups, whether online or in-person, can significantly boost motivation for managing hypertension and reduce feelings of isolation.

<u>Emotional Support</u>: Being diagnosed with hypertension can bring fear, confusion, and anxiety. Support groups create a space where members can express their concerns, share personal stories, and get reassurance from others who are going through similar challenges. Individuals in hypertension support groups experienced reduced stress levels, which in turn positively affected their blood pressure control.

<u>Shared Experiences</u>: When you connect with others who have similar experiences, it helps normalize the situation. You will hear firsthand strategies for dealing with high blood pressure, dietary tips, or coping mechanisms for managing stress. The value of shared

knowledge and lived experience cannot be overstated. People who actively engage in hypertension support groups report higher adherence to prescribed treatment plans and are more confident in managing their condition.

Types of Support Groups

Support comes in many forms, and finding the right group that meets your needs is crucial. From traditional face-to-face meetings to online platforms offering convenience and anonymity, different types of support groups can cater to your personal preferences and lifestyle.

<u>In-Person Groups</u>: These groups often meet in community centers, hospitals, or local organizations, allowing people to interact face-to-face. This personal interaction creates stronger bonds and fosters a sense of belonging. In-person groups typically have health professionals or experienced patients leading the discussion, providing not only peer support but also expert guidance. Such local groups also promote regular accountability, which can lead to better management of lifestyle choices and medication adherence.

<u>Online Communities</u>: <u>Online Forums, Social Media Platforms, and Virtual Meeting Groups</u> have become increasingly popular, especially for those who may not have access to local support groups or prefer the flexibility of digital communication. Platforms such as <u>Facebook Groups</u> or dedicated health forums offer 24/7 support, where members can post questions, share updates, and offer encouragement. Online groups are important for individuals who value anonymity, allowing them to share personal details without fear of judgment.

Specialized Groups: Some support groups cater to individuals with specific needs, such as those with secondary hypertension (where high blood pressure is caused by another medical condition) or those with additional chronic conditions like diabetes. These specialized groups ensure that discussions and shared experiences are tailored to unique health circumstances. Such specialized groups are particularly effective in addressing the complex medical regimens that patients with multiple conditions often face.

How to Find Support Groups

Finding the right support group can make a huge difference in your hypertension journey. Here are a few practical ways to locate a group that works for you:

Resources: Your healthcare provider or local hospital may offer information on support groups available in your area. Many hospitals run group meetings led by health professionals, which combine education with peer support. National health organizations, such as the American Heart Association (**AHA**), often maintain directories of support services and groups for hypertension patients.

Directories and Platforms: Online platforms such as *Meetup, Facebook Groups*, and dedicated health forums are excellent starting points for finding both local and virtual support groups. A simple online search for *"Hypertension Support Group"* in your area or joining general hypertension discussions can lead you to a community of like-minded individuals.

Educational Resources

Books, Websites, and Organizations for Further Reading

Staying well-informed about hypertension is one of the best ways to take control of your health. Reliable resources, including books, websites, and organizations, provide the latest research and practical advice that will empower you in your hypertension management.

Books

There is a wealth of literature available on managing high blood pressure. The following are some of the best, most accessible reads for anyone looking to deepen their understanding of hypertension:

"The Blood Pressure Solution" by Dr. Marlene Merritt: This comprehensive guide offers natural strategies for lowering blood pressure, alongside practical advice on diet, exercise, and stress management (Merritt, 2023).

"Hypertension: A Practical Guide" by Dr. V. K. Sahasranam: Known for its clear explanations, this book covers everything from the causes of hypertension to advanced treatment options, with a focus on empowering patients to make informed choices about their care.

"DASH diet for Dummies". Sarah Samaan, Rosanne Rust, Cindy Kleckner 2nd edition, John Wiley & sones. 2021.

"High Blood Pressure for Dummies". Richard W Snyder, Alan L Rubin. 3rd Edition Published by John Wiley & Sons. 2024.

"Mayo Clinic on High Blood Pressure" by Gary l Schwartz. Mayo Clinic Press. 2023.

Websites

For quick access to trusted, up-to-date information, the following websites provide a wealth of reliable resources:

- *American Heart Association* (**AHA**): This authoritative source offers everything from patient education materials to guidelines on hypertension management. You can find practical tips, research updates, and interactive tools like heart health risk calculators.
- *Centers for Disease Control and Prevention* (**CDC**): Known for its public health expertise, the CDC offers easy-to-understand information on hypertension prevention, management, and statistics.
- *National Heart, Lung, and Blood Institute* (**NHLBI**): This site provides educational materials, clinical guidelines, and a range of resources to help you understand the risks and management strategies associated with hypertension.

Organizations

Several organizations are dedicated to supporting those living with hypertension through advocacy, research, and education:

American Heart Association (**AHA**): A global leader in cardiovascular research and patient advocacy, the AHA provides support to individuals affected by high blood pressure through various programs and community resources.

American College of Cardiology (**ACC**):   Known for setting clinical guidelines, the ACC also offers resources aimed at helping patients manage their cardiovascular health.

For local support, check with community health organizations, regional hospitals, or patient advocacy foundations in your area.

How to Advocate for Yourself

Tips on Being an Informed and Proactive Patient

Being diagnosed with hypertension does not mean you should simply follow a doctor's orders passively. Advocating for yourself means being informed, asking questions, and taking an active role in managing your condition.

Education and Awareness

Understanding Your Condition: Knowledge is power when it comes to health. Take the time to understand what hypertension is, its risk factors, and the impact it has on your body. Make sure to read up on your medications and know how they work. Patients who actively educate themselves are better equipped to make decisions about their care.

Staying Updated: Research in the field of hypertension is constantly evolving. Stay updated on the latest treatment guidelines, medication options, and lifestyle strategies that can help manage your blood pressure. Subscribe to newsletters from reputable health organizations like the AHA to keep up with the latest developments.

<u>Effective Communication with Healthcare Providers</u>: Before each doctor's visit, prepare a list of questions or concerns. Do not hesitate to ask for clarification on anything you do not understand. Discuss your symptoms openly and honestly, as this helps healthcare providers tailor their recommendations to your needs.

Do not be afraid to voice your opinion when it comes to treatment decisions. If a prescribed treatment does not feel right, discuss alternatives with your doctor. Seeking second opinions is also encouraged if you are unsure about your current care plan.

<u>Self-Monitoring and Record Keeping</u>: Regularly monitor your blood pressure and maintain a health journal to track your readings, medication usage, and symptoms. This record can provide invaluable insight during doctor appointments and help adjust your treatment plan as necessary.

Blood pressure monitoring apps and wearable devices have made it easier than ever to track your blood pressure over time. The AHA offers resources to help you choose the right monitoring tools for your needs.

Advocacy and Resources

<u>Joining Advocacy Groups</u>: Advocacy groups not only support individuals with hypertension but also work to influence public policy and healthcare practices.

Joining these groups allows you to contribute to larger efforts in raising awareness and supporting research.

<u>Navigating Healthcare Systems</u>: Understanding your rights within healthcare systems and insurance plans can be challenging. The CDC provides valuable resources to help you navigate insurance, access necessary treatments, and ensure you're receiving adequate care.

Taking control of your hypertension management is a lifelong journey, but you do not have to do it alone. By finding support, educating yourself, and advocating for your health, you can live a full, empowered life despite your diagnosis. Remember: *You are your best advocate.*

More Resources

National Heart Lung and Blood Institute.

www.nhlbi.nih.gov

www.nhlbi.nih.gov/health

National kidney foundation

www.kidney.org

National institute of Diabetes and Digestive and Kidney diseases

www.niddk.nih.gov

American Heart and Stroke Associations

www.stroke.org   ASA

www.heart.org   AHA

National Library of Medicine

www.nlm.nih.gov

Medline plus

https://medlineplus.gov

https://medline plus.gov/highbloodpressure.html

provides medical encyclopedia, prescription and non pres drugs, Health info, Links to clinical trial, Lists of hospital and physicians by state.

PubMed

www.pubmed.gov

Mayo Clinic

www.mayoclinic.org

mayoclinic.org/diseases-conditions

American College of Lifestyle Medicine

https://lifestylemedicine.org/patient

www.lifestylemedpros.org

Centers for Disease control and Prevention

www.cdc.gov/bloodpressure

Key Takeaways

- *Support groups provide emotional and practical support, helping individuals with hypertension manage their condition more effectively.*

- *In-person and online communities offer different types of support, with online groups providing accessibility and anonymity for those unable to attend local meetings.*
- *Educational resources such as Books, Websites, and Organizations offer reliable, up-to-date information to help you stay informed about hypertension management.*
- *Advocating for yourself involves understanding your condition, asking the right questions, and actively participating in your treatment decisions.*
- *Self-monitoring through regular blood pressure tracking and using technology can help you stay on top of your health and share accurate data with healthcare providers.*
- *Joining advocacy groups and staying informed about the latest research empowers you to take an active role in managing hypertension and contributing to larger healthcare improvements.*

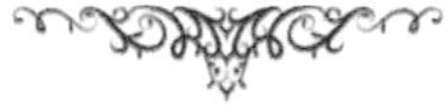

Chapter 21 - FUTURE DIRECTIONS IN HYPERTENSION RESEARCH AND TREATMENT

Hypertension research and treatment are advancing rapidly, offering new hope for more effective and personalized care. This chapter explores the future of hypertension management, highlighting emerging therapies, innovative technologies, and cutting-edge research. From new drug classes and gene-based treatments to wearable devices and artificial intelligence, the latest developments promise to revolutionize how we prevent and treat high blood pressure. As these innovations unfold, patients will benefit from more precise, convenient, and effective options for controlling their condition.

As the prevalence of hypertension continues to rise globally, the demand for new and effective treatments is becoming increasingly urgent. Fortunately, research into hypertension is advancing rapidly, with groundbreaking therapies, technologies, and innovations on the horizon. Let us explore the future of hypertension treatment, focusing on emerging drug therapies, technological advancements, and ongoing research. Understanding where hypertension management is headed will empower patients and healthcare providers to make more informed decisions as new options become available.

Emerging Therapies:

What is on the Horizon for Hypertension Treatment

Over the past few decades, several classes of antihypertensive medications have been developed. While these drugs have been effective in controlling blood pressure for millions of people, ongoing research is uncovering new treatment avenues. Novel therapies, including the development of new drug classes, combination treatments, and gene-based approaches, are poised to revolutionize the way we treat hypertension.

Novel Drug Classes

One of the most exciting areas of development in hypertension treatment is the emergence of new drug classes that target the condition from different angles.

Angiotensin Receptor Neprilysin Inhibitors (**ARNIs**): ARNIs are a relatively new class of drugs that combine an angiotensin receptor blocker (**ARB**) which helps relax blood vessels with another medication - *Neprilysin Inhibitor* which enhances the effects of natural substances in the body that lower blood pressure. Neprilysin is a substance that breaks down certain compounds, which help regulate blood pressure. By inhibiting neprilysin and blocking the angiotensin receptor, ARNIs both lower blood pressure and provide cardiovascular benefits. ARNIs show significant promise in controlling hypertension, particularly in patients who are not responding well to conventional treatments. These have been found to be immensely helpful particularly in heart failure. It is available in the market.

Renin Inhibitors: Another emerging class involves direct renin inhibitors, which target the enzyme *Renin*, a key player in the regulation of blood pressure. *Aliskiren*, a renin inhibitor, has shown positive results in lowering blood pressure but is still under study for broader use. It is effective as part of combination therapy for resistant hypertension.

Combination Therapies

The concept of combining multiple antihypertensive agents into a single treatment has gained traction as a way to improve patient adherence and enhance blood pressure control.

Fixed-Dose Combinations: Fixed-dose combinations (**FDCs**) involve combining two or more antihypertensive drugs into a single pill. This simplifies the treatment regimen for patients and reduces the likelihood of missed doses. The growing popularity of

FDCs in hypertension treatment, with studies showing improved blood pressure control and better compliance is now accepted. These combinations are already available freely in countries like India and often the combination is cheaper than the individual drugs.

<u>Personalized Medicine</u>: Advances in genetic research have paved the way for personalized medicine, where treatment plans are tailored to the individual based on their genetic makeup and response to drugs. In the near future, hypertensive patients will undergo genetic testing to determine the most effective drug combinations for their specific condition, leading to more precise and effective treatment.

Biological and Gene-Based Therapies

In addition to drug-based treatments, the future of hypertension management may also include therapies that target the underlying genetic and biological causes of high blood pressure.

<u>Gene Therapy</u>: Gene-editing technologies are being explored as potential treatments for hypertension by addressing the genetic causes of the disease. While this area is still in its infancy, Gene therapy could one day offer a long-term solution for patients with hypertension caused by specific genetic mutations.

<u>Biologics</u>: Monoclonal antibodies and other biologic treatments are being developed to target specific molecular pathways involved in hypertension. Monoclonal antibodies are clones of the body's natural antibodies that are made in a laboratory. These are meant to stimulate the immune system. Biologics offer a novel approach to hypertension treatment by addressing

the underlying biology of the disease, particularly in cases of drug-resistant hypertension.

Technological Advances

Technology is rapidly transforming the way we monitor and manage hypertension. From wearable devices that provide real-time data to telemedicine platforms that offer remote consultations, these advancements are making hypertension management more accessible, efficient, and personalized.

Wearable Devices

Wearable technology has made significant strides in recent years, and the integration of blood pressure monitoring into devices like smartwatches and fitness trackers is already changing how people track their health.

Smartwatches and Fitness Trackers: Many modern smartwatches now include blood pressure monitoring features, allowing users to check their blood pressure anytime, anywhere. These devices not only provide convenience but also enable continuous monitoring, which can help detect patterns and fluctuations in blood pressure throughout the day. Wearable technology could lead to earlier detection of hypertension and better long-term management.

Advanced Sensors: New developments in sensor technology are enabling non-invasive, real-time blood pressure monitoring. The potential of these sensors to revolutionize hypertension management by providing more accurate and frequent blood pressure readings without the need for traditional cuffs is being recognized.

Telemedicine and Remote Monitoring

Telemedicine is playing an increasingly important role in healthcare, and hypertension management is no exception. Remote monitoring allows patients to track their blood pressure from home and share the data with healthcare providers in real-time.

Telehealth Platforms: Telemedicine platforms offer patients the convenience of consulting with their doctors from home, making healthcare more accessible, especially for those in remote areas. Telemedicine has been particularly effective in managing hypertension, as it allows for frequent follow-ups and adjustments to treatment plans without the need for in-person visits.

Data Integration: The integration of home blood pressure monitoring data with electronic health records (**EHRs**) is a game-changer in hypertension management. By automatically syncing patient data with their healthcare provider's system, doctors can make more informed decisions and track patient progress more effectively. Data integration improves patient outcomes by enabling real-time monitoring and personalized treatment adjustments.

Artificial Intelligence and Machine Learning

Artificial intelligence (**AI**) and machine learning are becoming valuable tools in predicting and managing hypertension.

Predictive Analytics: AI-driven models can analyze large datasets to predict blood pressure trends and assess the risk of developing hypertension. Predictive models are helping doctors identify patients at risk earlier, allowing for preventive measures to be taken before hypertension becomes a serious issue.

Decision Support Systems: AI-based decision support systems are being developed to assist clinicians in personalizing hypertension treatment plans. These systems analyze patient data and recommend the most effective treatment options, taking into account factors such as genetic markers, lifestyle, and medication response. These tools have the potential to revolutionize personalized care in hypertension.

Research and Innovations:

Ongoing research into the genetic and molecular basis of hypertension is leading to exciting discoveries that could reshape treatment strategies. Innovations such as pharmacogenomics, stem cell research, and advanced drug delivery systems are opening new doors for more effective and personalized hypertension care.

Pharmacogenomics

Pharmacogenomics is the study of how genes affect a person's response to drugs, and it holds great promise for hypertension treatment.

Genetic Variability: Researchers are studying how genetic differences influence individual responses to antihypertensive medications. Understanding these genetic factors can lead to more effective and personalized treatment plans, reducing the trial-and-error approach currently used in prescribing hypertension medications.

Personalized Dosing: As pharmacogenomics research progresses, doctors may soon be able to tailor not only the type of medication but also the dosage based on a patient's genetic profile. Personalized dosing could significantly improve blood pressure control while minimizing side effects.

Stem Cell Research

Stem cell therapy is an exciting area of research that may offer new solutions for managing hypertension and repairing cardiovascular damage.

Regenerative Medicine: Stem cells have the potential to regenerate damaged blood vessels and heart tissue, offering a new approach to treating hypertension-related complications. It is being investigated how stem cell therapies could be used to repair the cardiovascular damage caused by chronic hypertension, potentially reducing the need for long-term medication.

Ongoing clinical trials are exploring the safety and efficacy of stem cell therapies for severe hypertension and related conditions. Early results are promising, though more research is needed before these treatments become widely available.

Innovative Drug Delivery Systems

In addition to developing new drugs, researchers are also focusing on improving how existing medications are delivered to the body.

Nanotechnology: Nanocarriers, which are tiny particles designed to deliver drugs directly to specific cells or tissues, are being studied as a way to improve the efficacy of hypertension treatments. Nanotechnology could enable more targeted drug delivery, reducing side effects and improving therapeutic outcomes.

Long-Acting Formulations: Long-acting drug formulations are being developed to improve patient adherence and provide more consistent blood pressure control. These formulations could reduce the frequency of doses, making it easier for patients to stick to their treatment regimens.

The future of hypertension treatment is bright, with new therapies, technologies, and research promising to transform the way we manage high blood pressure. From novel drug classes and wearable technology to AI-driven tools and personalized medicine, these advancements offer hope for more effective and individualized care. As research continues to push the boundaries of what is possible, patients and healthcare providers alike will benefit from these innovative approaches.

Key Takeaways

- *New drug classes, such as Angiotensin Receptor Neprilysin Inhibitors (ARNIs) and renin inhibitors, are showing promise in improving hypertension management.*
- *Fixed-dose combination therapies simplify treatment by combining multiple medications in one pill, improving adherence and blood pressure control.*

- *Personalized medicine is emerging, using genetic profiles to tailor hypertension treatments for better outcomes.*
- *Wearable devices like smartwatches are integrating blood pressure monitoring, offering real-time data for more effective hypertension management.*
- *Telemedicine and remote monitoring make hypertension care more accessible, allowing for regular tracking and virtual consultations.*
- *Artificial intelligence is being used to predict blood pressure trends and assist clinicians in personalizing treatment plans.*
- *Pharmacogenomics and stem cell research are paving the way for personalized and regenerative approaches to hypertension care.*
- *Innovative drug delivery systems, including nanotechnology and long-acting formulations, are improving the efficacy and convenience of hypertension treatment.*

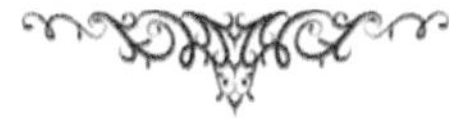

Resources & References

Books

1. *"DASH diet for Dummies"*: Sarah Samaan, Rosanne Rust, Cindy Kleckner 2nd edition, John Wiley & sones. 2021.
2. *"High Blood Pressure for Dummies"*: Richard W Snyder, Alan L Rubin
   3rd Edition Published by John Wiley & Sons. 2024.
3. *"Mayo Clinic on High Blood Pressure"*: by Gary l Schwartz. Mayo Clinic Press. 2023
4. *"Davidson's Principle and Practice of Medicine"*: Ed. Ralston SH et al. 23rd Edition, Elsevier 2018.
5. Systemic Hypertension: Mechanisms and Diagnosis: Ronald G Victor. In *Braunwald's Heart Disease*. Vol II. Edited by Mann DL, Zipes DP, Libby P, Bonow RO. 10th Edition. 2015
6. Systemic Hypertension: Management: Ronald G Victor & Peter Libby. In *Braunwald's Heart Disease*. Vol II. Edited by Mann DL, Zipes DP, Libby P, Bonow RO. 10th Edition. 2015

References

1. A new immune disease : Systemic Hypertension.

https://academic.oup.com/ckj/article/16/9/1403/7085
012

2. Alcohol intake and risk of Hypertension.

https://www.ahajournals.org/doi/full/10.1161/HYPER
TENSIONAHA.124.22703#:~:text=The%20increased%
20risk%20of%20hypertension,content%20in%20the%2
0following%20formats:

3. New drug strategies for treating Hypertension

https://link.springer.com/article/10.1007/s40292-024-
00634-4

4. Systematic Review Hypertension

https://www.ncbi.nlm.nih.gov/pmc/articles/PMC10518
047/

5. Management of Hypertension in acute care setting
    2024 -AHA

https://www.ahajournals.org/doi/10.1161/HYP.00000
00000000238

6. Hypertension control rate in India   Lancet

https://www.thelancet.com/journals/lansea/article/PII
S2772-3682(22)00130-5/fulltext

7. Systemic Hypertension 2022

https://www.healthline.com/health/high-blood-
pressure-hypertension/systemic-
hypertension#symptoms

8. Hypertension: Medscape 2024

https://emedicine.medscape.com/article/241381-overview?form=fpf

9. Treatment of Hypertension: Review   2019

https://www.scirp.org/journal/paperinformation?paperid=91358

10. Hypertension : WHO 2023

https://www.who.int/news-room/fact-sheets/detail/hypertension

11. Hypertension : Mayo clinic

https://www.mayoclinic.org/diseases-conditions/high-blood-pressure/symptoms-causes/syc-20373410

12. Hypertension : Wikipedia

https://en.wikipedia.org/wiki/Hypertension

13. High Blood Pressure. Diagnosis and treatment: Mayo clinic

https://www.mayoclinic.org/diseases-conditions/high-blood-pressure/diagnosis-treatment/drc-20373417

14. What to know about Primary Hypertension : Cleveland clinic

https://my.clevelandclinic.org/health/diseases/22024-primary-hypertension-formerly-known-as-essential-hypertension

15. European Society of Cardiology Guidelines in Hypertension : 2024

https://academic.oup.com/eurheartj/advance-article/doi/10.1093/eurheartj/ehae178/7741010

16. High Blood pressure : American Heart Association.

https://www.heart.org/en/health-topics/high-blood-pressure

17. Blood Pressure target in adults : Family Practice Guidelines – 2022

https://www.aafp.org/dam/AAFP/documents/journals/afp/AAFPHypertensionGuideline.pdf

18. History of Hypertension : Wikipedia

https://en.wikipedia.org/wiki/History_of_hypertension

19. Historical trends in Hypertension research: AHA 2011

https://www.ahajournals.org/doi/10.1161/HYPERTENSIONAHA.111.177766

20. Ambulatory Blood Pressure monitoring: CSI Article K V Sahasranam.
21. Goal blood pressure in adults with hypertension: Johannes FE Mann, Karl F Hilgers, UpToDate Aug. 2024.
22. Labile Hypertension : Samuel J Mann. UpToDate Aug 2024.
23. Management of severe asymptomatic hypertension (hypertensive urgencies) in adults: Joseph Varon, William J Elliott, UpToDate Aug 2024.
24. Treatment of hypertension in pregnant and postpartum patients: Phyllis August UpToDate Aug 2024.

25. Evaluation Of Secondary Hypertension: William B White UpToDate Aug 2024

26. Treatment Of Hypertension In Older Adults, Particularly Isolated Systolic Hypertension. Brent M Egan, UpToDate Aug 2024

27. Initial Management Of Hypertensive Emergencies And Urgencies In Children: Joseph T Flynn UpToDate Aug 2024

28. Hypertensive Disorders In Pregnancy: Approach To Differential Diagnosis: Phyllis August, Baha M Sibai. UpToDate Aug 2024

29. Hypertension In Children And Adolescents: Nonemergency Treatment: Tej K Mattoo UpToDate Aug 2024

30. Hypertension In Children And Adolescents: Epidemiology, Risk Factors, And Etiology: Tej K Mattoo Aug 2024.

Acknowledgement

I owe immense gratitude to my family for their unwavering support throughout the process of writing this book. Their encouragement has been invaluable. My daughter, Sandya, has been especially helpful, guiding me through the nuances of computer use and assisting with the text formatting and preparation of the QR codes for my books.

My sincere gratitude goes to Prof. R. Krishnan, Senior Physician at Baby Memorial Hospital, Calicut, who generously provided me with invaluable references and resources essential for the creation of this book.

I am also deeply thankful to my colleagues in the author community, who generously assisted me and provided constructive feedback on my previous works. They have been quick to offer advice whenever I faced challenges in my writing.

Special recognition goes to Mr. Som Bathla, my mentor on this journey, and to the members of the Author-Helping-Author (AHA) community, whose guidance has been instrumental in shaping my writing and publishing endeavors.

My teachers in the medical schools where I received my undergraduate and postgraduate training deserve special mention. I have achieved what I have by standing on the shoulders of these giants who taught me the art and science of medicine. My deepest respect and gratitude go to them.

I thank depositphotos.com for the beautiful pictures of the heart and other figures included in this book.